ANATOMY™
OF FITNESS

Yoga

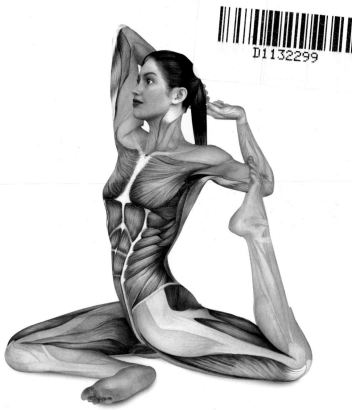

hinkler

Created by Moseley Road Inc.
Editorial director: Lisa Purcell
Art director: Brian MacMullen
Cover and internals designer: Sam Grimmer
Photographer: Jonathan Conklin Photography, Inc.
Author: Goldie Karpel Oren
Model: Lana Russo
Illustrator: Hector Aiza/3DLabz
Prepress: Graphic Print Group
Inset illustrations © Linda Bucklin/Shutterstock.com,
page 5 © heaven/Shutterstock.com,
page 6 © Ekaterina Garyuk/Shutterstock.com,
page 7 top © Brooke Becker/Shutterstock.com,
page 7 bottom © StockLite/Shutterstock.com,
page 9 © zhuda/Shutterstock.com

Contents

Yoga: Mind & Body Fitness

The practice of yoga not only disciplines your body, but also helps to discipline your mind.

Yoga is more than just another form of fitness: the practice transcends the physicality of its postures. Yoga is also a mental and spiritual practice, in the sense that the work that goes into aligning the body can also be used to align your mind.

In yoga we are trying to calm the fluctuations of the mind. Our minds have a tendency to think in past and future tenses. In yoga, we have to concentrate on keeping our thoughts in the present moment. You will find, by practicing this technique, that you are more fully present on a daily basis.

This book contains a well-balanced, flowing sequence of poses. You will build strength and flexibility while improving your concentration and willpower. You will learn to control your body

with your mind and come to understand that, as in life, with time and patience you can overcome many obstacles.

You will see, for example, that your mind will want to give up before your body needs to come out of a pose; you'll learn to understand the distinction between pain and discomfort. If you suffer actual pain from an injury then you should come out of a pose, but otherwise, try to breathe through any discomfort.

Sometimes you will have intense sensations in your muscles—it is normal to have these feelings while holding a yoga pose. Sometimes we have to ignore what our minds are telling us and move beyond thinking, "I can't hold this any longer." *Your body is strong enough to hold the posture for longer than you think.* By holding a yoga pose for a

Challenge yourself

Your breath will get you through the demanding poses. For instance, challenge yourself to hold Plank Pose (pages 28–29) for one or even two minutes, which is about 10 to 20 long, deep breath cycles. Not only will you build core strength, but you will also cultivate internal strength, stamina, and willpower. Stay in the position longer than you want to. Finding stillness of the body and stillness of the mind is the most challenging aspect of yoga. Holding the poses is often more difficult than moving and flowing.

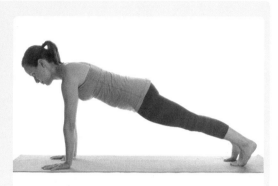

few extra breaths, you will begin to build inner strength. You will learn that you are stronger than you imagined.

In the world we live in, we are used to instant gratification. By practicing yoga and holding the poses, which can be uncomfortable, you will build patience. You will find that you can take a step back, pause, and breathe. You will find that turning off your phone for an hour and rolling out your mat can be quite rewarding. You will know, when you finish with your practice, that you can take an hour to shut out your to-do lists and distracting thoughts, following through on an important decision to focus on your breath and the alignment of your body.

You will be able to use lessons learned on the yoga mat in your daily life, knowing that no challenging situation will last forever, just as no yoga posture lasts forever. Yoga teaches us to be completely present in every moment of our lives, whether it is

a good time or a bad one. Stress is often brought on by worrying about the future, or by dwelling on events in the past. The stress that you experience may be caused by the thoughts in your head—the situation you are in may not actually be too stressful after all. With your yoga practice, you will see that by changing how you think about things, you can change your outlook. So give yourself that extra moment to pause and take a deep breath.

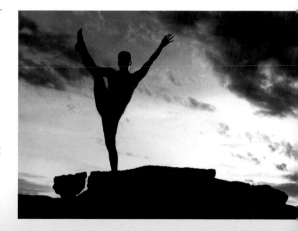

Home Practice

To get the most out of your yoga practice, dedicate a particular area within your home as your yoga space. This is where you should practice on a regular schedule.

The greatest challenge of practicing yoga at home, rather than at a studio, is learning to shut out all potential distractions. Your family, phones, computer, and television can prevent you from concentrating on what you are doing. When practicing at home, you need to create a space in which you can block out those distractions. Designate a room or area where you will always practice. Make a schedule for yourself, setting aside perhaps 30 minutes at the same time every day, five days a week. The great thing about yoga is that you don't need a lot of space—just the length of the yoga mat. When traveling, you can pack your mat in your suitcase and roll it out wherever you are.

Equipment and clothing

To begin your home practice, you will need a yoga block, a yoga strap, and a yoga mat. A block aids you during standing poses that call for you to place a hand on the floor. A strap helps you to achieve a full stretch. And you don't need specially designed yoga equipment: a book will easily stand in for a yoga block, and a long belt or sash will work just as well as a yoga strap. A yoga mat is different from a Pilates mat or a padded gym mat. Buy a mat specifically designed for yoga that is thin and sticky, so that you have the traction to grip the floor with your hands and feet. Wear a comfortable top and pants, and leave off the socks. Practicing barefoot will help you to ground your hands and feet into the floor.

Flexibility and body awareness

Everyone has a different level of natural flexibility; strength and flexibility are two traits that, as humans, we need to work on constantly. Don't feel that you can't take a yoga class because you're not flexible! This is why we call yoga a "practice." Each individual has a tendency toward either being more flexible or having tighter muscles, and in yoga we're trying to find that balance between our strength

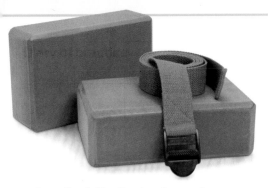

and our flexibility. Our bodies and minds are constantly changing and evolving—every time you come to your mat you will feel different than you felt the last time you did yoga. This is what makes the yoga practice interesting. We may perform the same poses time and time again, yet each time we find something new to work on. An advanced practitioner is not necessarily someone who can come into the most challenging pose; being advanced means having the body awareness and control to work the subtleties of each pose.

Using your tools

Think of your yoga props as tools to help you deepen your poses. Don't think that using the block and strap makes you a "beginner," or that you're not really doing the pose if you use them. In Extended Triangle with Block (pages 36–37), for example, the point of the pose is not to reach your palms to the floor; the goal is to elongate your spine, finding length on all four sides of your torso. If your hand is on the floor but the side of your body is crunched and you can't breathe, then you're not doing yoga—you are just contorting your body. Instead, use your block to your advantage, and create the space you need to deepen your breath.

Dedicated space

There's no need to call in a carpenter to build you a home yoga studio. Your goal is to simply reserve a quiet space within your home—a space in which to retreat regularly to practice yoga.

If you live in a large house, you may have the luxury of transforming an entire room into a private yoga studio. But if your space is smaller, you can still create a peaceful sanctuary. Just designate an area large enough to stretch fully and lunge freely, without obstructions. A movable screen, such as a folding Shoji screen, can lend privacy, as can curtains or drapery that you can easily open and close.

Store your yoga mat, blocks, straps, and other gear within this space for easy access, and don't forget the atmosphere-setting extras. Gather things that inspire you: plants, stones, and other natural objects can set the mood. A swirling image that you can meditate on or a flickering candle for your eyes to lock onto while you hold that pose just a few breaths longer can add greatly to your yoga practice.

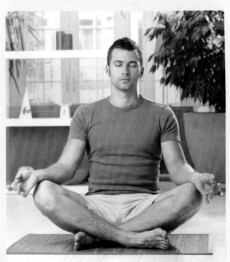

Breath Control

We may take breathing—the very essence of life—for granted, but learning how to do it properly and mindfully will enhance your yoga practice.

Your breath will guide you through your practice. The style of the sequence in this book is that of a Vinyasa flow class. The word *vinyasa* means "to link" or "to connect." In your practice you are linking your breath with your movement, and your movement with your breath. You will

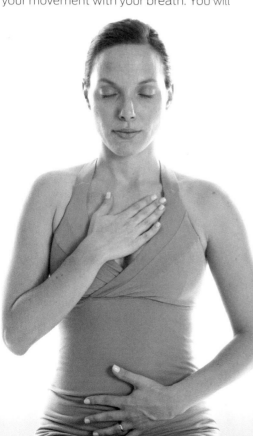

begin to create a moving meditation. As you hold the poses and flow from one to the next, you'll focus on lengthening and deepening your breath, and in this way yoga is simply a breathing exercise. If you find yourself holding your breath or breathing heavily, take a step back and re-evaluate your position. This may mean holding the pose for a shorter time, choosing a less challenging variation of the posture, or resting in Child's Pose (pages 14–15). Our minds constantly jump from thought to thought, focusing on situations and stories from the past and worrying about and planning the future, so that much of the time we forget to live in the present moment. The breath is our tool for staying in the present moment. By concentrating on our breath, we are forced to put aside any other thoughts that may be cluttering up our brains.

Pranayama

In Sanskrit, *prana* means "life force" or "energy," and *ayama* means "to control or extend." Together the two form the word *pranayama*, which means "extension of the life force," or "breath control." The practice of yoga calls for us to pay close attention to the process of breathing in and out, which we usually take for granted.

Kapalabhati

There are several ways to manipulate the breath. One of the most common methods of warm-up breathing is Kapalabhati. *Kapal* means "skull," and *bhati* means "shining"; together the two words mean "shining skull." This is a breathing technique that will cleanse your sinuses. In Kapalabhati, you control the breath by sharply exhaling while pumping your stomach in and out. The inhalation is passive, while the exhalation is forceful and sharp. The sharp and rapid exhales will help your lungs to clear any waste from your air passageways.

Ujjayi Pranayama

Another common breathing technique is Ujjayi Pranayama. This technique calms the brain and creates internal heat. When done correctly, Ujjayi sounds like the ocean, so it is often called "ocean breath." During the execution of Ujjayi Pranayama, your mouth stays closed, and there is a slight constriction of your throat as you inhale and exhale.

Because it is deep and mindful, the breath will help to calm your nervous system. This type of breath will help to reduce stress by stimulating the parasympathetic response of the central nervous system instead of the fight-or-flight response, which increases adrenaline. This relaxation response will help to quiet your mind, reduce stress, and make you feel good when you leave your mat.

Practicing Ujjayi

Proper breath is an essential element of yoga. Start by practicing Ujjayi Pranayama.

1 Begin by sitting up tall in a comfortable position, such as Easy Pose (pages 12–13).

2 Hold your hand in front of your mouth and imagine that your hand is a mirror. Open your mouth and exhale a *hah* sound, as if you were fogging up a mirror. That breath comes from the back of your throat.

3 Now close your mouth, and try to breathe in a similar way, as if you were fogging up that imaginary mirror. You will notice a hissing sound coming from the back of your throat. This is the start to practicing the Ujjayi breathing technique.

Practice about 8 to 10 breath cycles, inhaling and exhaling with this slight constriction at the back of your throat. As you begin to feel more comfortable, you will naturally start to breathe in this way throughout the entire vinyasa yoga practice. The Ujjayi technique will start to effortlessly flow from one breath to the next, helping you to connect your movement with your breath.

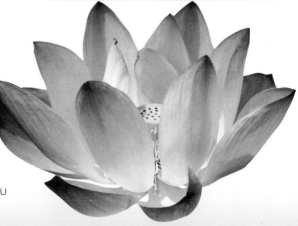

The Yoga Sequence

The following pages will guide you through a flowing sequence of poses that help to increase strength and flexibility while improving concentration and willpower.

The yoga sequence in this book consists of 23 individual yoga poses. Some of the poses will be repeated. For each pose, you will find step-by-step instructions as well as notes on correct form. You can make the practice your own by going at your own pace; if you like, you can stay in the poses longer than recommended, taking extra breaths where you need to.

How to practice the yoga sequence

Begin the yoga sequence by taking a seated position, with your eyes closed. Use this time to center yourself and bring your awareness to your breath.

From the seated position you will make your way into Downward-Facing Dog, a pose that you will come into often throughout the flow. You will go on to perform several Sun Salutation A's to build internal heat as you warm up. The Sun Salutations help you connect to your breath. The flowing sequence focuses the mind and synchronizes it with your body and breath, drawing you deeper into the practice. Each pose that forms part of the Sun Salutation A sequence is connected to a breath call, either an inhalation or an exhalation. The sequence flows smoothly from pose to pose, using the breath to help move you.

Terms to know

Certain terms that are often heard in a yoga class will appear throughout the book.

vinyasa: The word *vinyasa* literally means "to link or connect." In a yoga class it can also mean a specific sequence of breath-synchronized movements used to transition between sustained postures: Plank Pose, Chaturanga, Upward-Facing Dog, Downward-Facing Dog. The entire sequence of poses in this book can also be called "vinyasa" because you are linking your breath with your movement and your movement with your breath.

alignment: In the yoga practice each pose has an ideal position of the body. If the body is in alignment, then it is placed in a proper way so that the muscles can work more effectively; they don't have to grip or struggle to hold the position, thus preventing injury. Each pose has its own alignment points, such as where to place your hands, feet, or torso, so learning a pose means also learning its proper points of alignment.

heel-to-heel alignment: When your feet are separated wide apart, if you were draw a line from one foot to the other, the heels would be on the same line. This type of alignment is used when practicing internally rotated postures.

heel-to-arch alignment: When your feet are separated wide apart, if you were draw a line from your front foot, it would intersect with the inner arch of the back foot. This type of alignment is used in externally rotated postures.

internally rotate: The body part moves in toward the center of the body.

externally rotate: The body part moves away from the center of the body.

ground down: To press your hands or feet (foundation) into the floor.

energy up: Energy isn't tangible, but in the yoga practice you are moving stale energy around and trying to lift your energy levels. "Energy up" is a subtle feeling of an upward lift.

After Sun Salutation A you will hold several externally rotated standing positions, which will help to open your hips. Next, you will move into the internally rotated postures that form Sun Salutation B, either choosing to hold Chair or Warrior I, or flow through the sequence holding each pose in the sequence for one breath. After the standing postures you will practice backbends, often called "heart-openers." You'll then begin to cool down and calm your mind with several stretches and forward bends leading up to your final deep relaxation, called Savasana, or Corpse Pose.

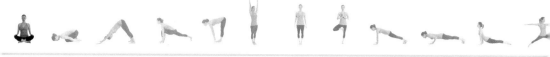

Easy Pose
(Sukhasana)

If your hamstrings, lower back, or hip flexors are tight then Easy Pose will not be so easy! As you continue to practice yoga, you will find the pose becoming more comfortable—and in time, you'll be able to sit and meditate for hours.

1 Sit on the floor, bend your knees, and cross your legs at the shins. Flex your feet to keep your knees in alignment. Feel both sitting bones firmly pressing into the floor and find a neutral pelvis. Lengthen your spine by sitting up straight and opening up across your collarbones.

2 Place your hands on your thighs with your palms facing either up or down.

3 Close your eyes and draw your focus inward. Lengthen your inhalation and exhalation, aiming for equal length. Try to match the length of your exhale to your inhale. Hold this pose for 5 to 10 breaths.

4 Easy Pose is a common position used for Pranayama and meditation. Close your eyes and draw your focus inward. You can begin by simply lengthening your inhalation and lengthening your exhalation. Try to match the length of your exhale to your inhale. Hold this pose for 1 to 3 minutes.

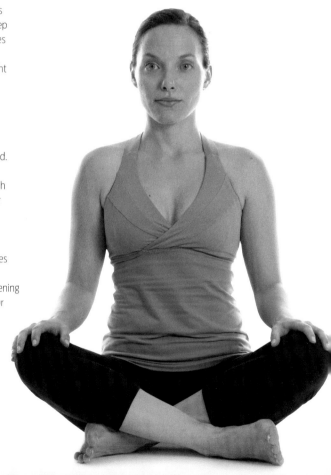

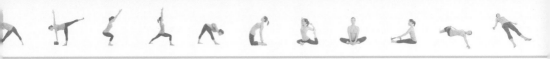

Diary of practice

	Date	No. of Breaths	Comment
Week 1			
Week 2			
Week 3			
Week 4			

Correct form
· Sit on a block or blanket to elevate your hips above the level of your knees.
· Alternate the crossing of your shins. We all have a dominant side; allow your less dominant side to stretch and find balance in the hips by switching the crossing of your shins.

Avoid
· Letting your knees rise above your hips.
· Rounding your shoulders.

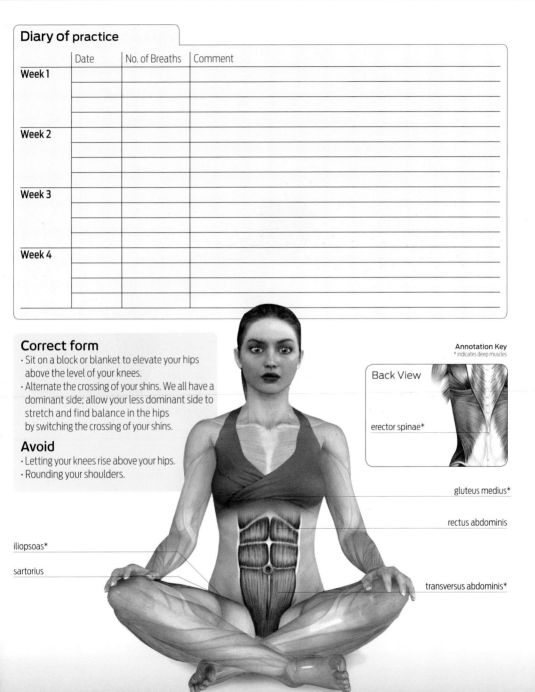

Annotation Key
* indicates deep muscles

Back View

erector spinae*

gluteus medius*

rectus abdominis

iliopsoas*

sartorius

transversus abdominis*

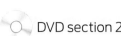

🔘 DVD section 2: Chapter 2

Child's Pose
(Balasana)

Very relaxing and restorative, Child's Pose is a perfect resting position that you can assume at any point during your practice.

1 From Easy Pose (pages 12–13), uncross your legs and come onto your hands and knees.

2 Bring your big toes together and your knees about hip-distance apart.

3 Sit your hips back onto your heels as you extend your torso forward, laying your stomach onto your thighs. Let your shoulders round forward, allowing your forehead to rest gently on the floor.

4 Bring your arms by your sides with the palms of your hands facing upward. Breathe into the back of your body. Hold for 5 to 10 breaths.

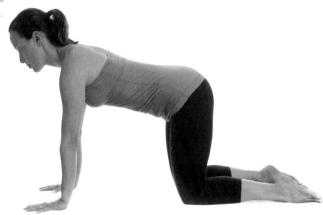

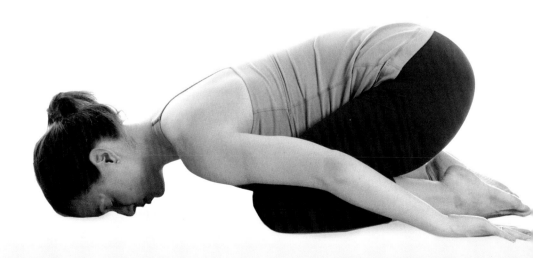

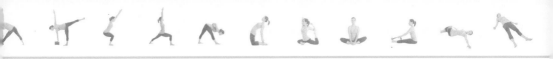

Diary of practice

	Date	No. of Breaths	Comment
Week 1			
Week 2			
Week 3			
Week 4			

Correct form
· Relax any tension you are holding in your jaw and face muscles.
· Open up between your shoulder blades as you breathe.

Avoid
· Bringing your knees too far apart.

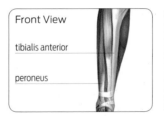

Front View

tibialis anterior

peroneus

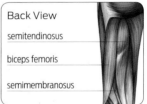

Back View

semitendinosus

biceps femoris

semimembranosus

Annotation Key
* indicates deep muscles

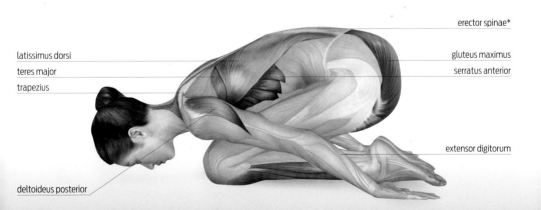

erector spinae*

latissimus dorsi

teres major

trapezius

gluteus maximus

serratus anterior

extensor digitorum

deltoideus posterior

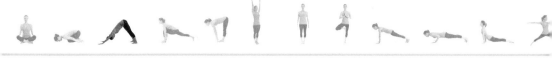

 DVD section 2: Chapter 3

Downward-Facing Dog
(Adho Mukha Svanasana)

Downward-Facing Dog is among the most frequently performed yoga poses—one you'll come into time and again. "Down Dog," as it is often known, stretches and strengthens the entire body. Because your head is below your heart in this pose, it is known as an "inversion."

1 From Child's Pose (pages 14–15), come onto your hands and knees, with your hands aligned under your shoulders and your knees under your hips.

2 Tuck your toes under, and "walk" your hands forward about a palm's distance in front of your shoulders. With hands and toes planted, lift your hips up as you straighten your legs and draw your heels toward the floor.

Correct form
- If you have tight shoulders, plant your hands more widely, and if the backs of your legs are tight, plant your feet more widely.
- To find the correct foot position, lift your toes, spread them out, and lower them. Press evenly through your feet and draw your inner ankles up to lift your arches, and then bring your heels toward the floor.
- To focus on your arms and hands, line up your wrist creases parallel to the front of the mat, resist your forearms away from the floor, and externally rotate your outer upper arms, drawing your inner elbows forward. Spread your fingers wide and ground down through every knuckle. Keep your middle finger pointing forward.

Avoid
- Internally rotating your arms and sinking into your shoulders.
- Rounding or over-arching your lower back.
- Letting your front ribs jut forward.

3 Press your chest toward your thighs, and bring your head between your arms. Lengthen up through your tailbone and keep your thighs slightly internally rotated, finding a neutral pelvis. Gaze between your feet or toward your navel. Hold for 5 to 10 breaths.

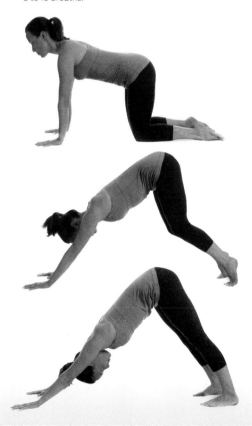

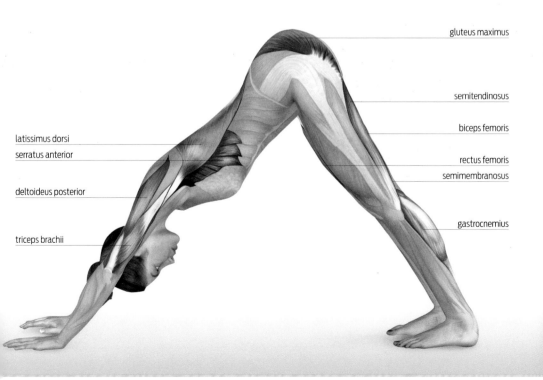

Diary of practice

	Date	No. of Breaths	Comment
Week 1			
Week 2			
Week 3			
Week 4			

gluteus maximus

semitendinosus

biceps femoris

latissimus dorsi

serratus anterior

rectus femoris

semimembranosus

deltoideus posterior

gastrocnemius

triceps brachii

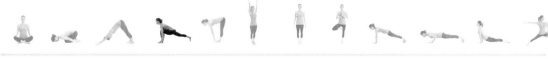

 DVD section 2: Chapter 4

High Lunge

High Lunge is a pose that can be held for several breaths or used as a transitional pose in the Sun Salutation sequences as a way to step back to Downward-Facing Dog or as a way to step forward into Standing Forward Bend.

1 From Downward-Facing Dog (pages 16–17), step your left foot forward in between your hands, with your left knee and shin lined up over your left ankle.

2 With your fingertips resting on the floor, square your hips to the front of the mat, grounding your left heel into the floor and drawing your left hip crease back.

3 Extend your right leg straight behind you, resting the ball of your foot on the mat. Lengthen all the way from the crown of your head to your right heel. Gaze slightly ahead, keeping the back of your neck long. Hold for 1 to 5 breaths. Later in the sequence, repeat on the other side.

Correct form
- Bring your belly in, away from your thigh.
- Keep your thighs firm as you stretch.
- Roll the inner thigh of your straight leg toward the ceiling, finding its internal rotation.
- If your back begins rounding when your fingertips touch the floor, bring your hands onto blocks to help elongate your spine.

Avoid
- Letting your stomach hang down.
- Positioning your knee past your ankle and over your toes, which can stress your knee joint.

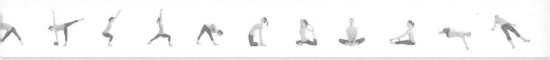

Diary of practice

	Date	No. of Breaths	Comment
Week 1			
Week 2			
Week 3			
Week 4			

Annotation Key
* indicates deep muscles

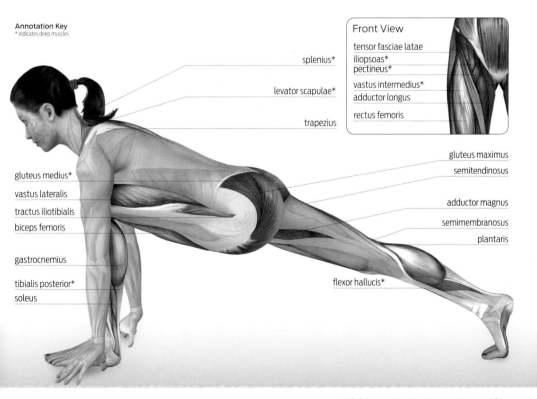

splenius*

levator scapulae*

trapezius

Front View

tensor fasciae latae
iliopsoas*
pectineus*
vastus intermedius*
adductor longus
rectus femoris

gluteus maximus

semitendinosus

adductor magnus

semimembranosus

plantaris

gluteus medius*

vastus lateralis

tractus iliotibialis

biceps femoris

gastrocnemius

tibialis posterior*

soleus

flexor hallucis*

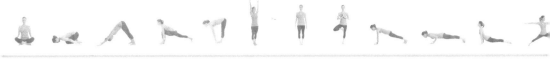

Standing Half Forward Bend to Standing Forward Bend
(Ardha Uttanasana to Uttanasana)

Often repeated throughout yoga classes, Standing Half Forward Bend and Standing Forward Bend form part of the Sun Salutation sequences. Each time you perform these poses, you will fold a little deeper into the forward bend.

1 From High Lunge (pages 18–19), inhale to step your back foot forward to meet your front foot. Spread out your toes and press down evenly through all four corners of your feet.

2 Plant your fingertips in line with your toes and look forward. Straighten your legs and arms as you lift your chest up away from your legs. Broaden across the front of your chest, finding a slight backward bend in your upper back as you draw your stomach in.

3 Press your heels into the floor as you lift your tailbone up toward the ceiling, keeping your hips in line with your heels. This is Standing Half Forward Bend.

4 Inhale to lengthen your spine, then exhale as you fold forward, hinging at the hips and bringing your fingertips or palms to the floor. This is Standing Forward Bend.

5 Lengthen your torso as you bring your belly closer to your thighs, ground your heels into the floor, and lift your tailbone toward the ceiling. Hold for 1 to 5 breaths, inhaling to lengthen the spine and exhaling to fold deeper.

Correct form
- Keep a slight bend in your knees if you have a tight lower back or hamstrings. Separating your feet hip-width apart also helps if you have tight hamstrings.
- If you can't reach the floor during Standing Half Forward Bend, place your hands on your shins.
- If you cannot reach the floor during Standing Forward Bend, place your hands on blocks or bend your arms and hold opposite elbows.

Avoid
- Shifting your weight backward so that your hips are behind your heels.

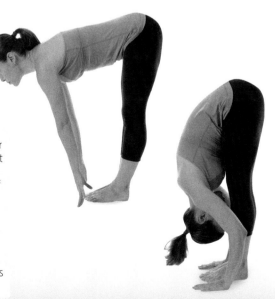

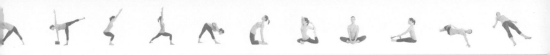

	Date	No. of Breaths	Comment
Week 1			
Week 2			
Week 3			
Week 4			

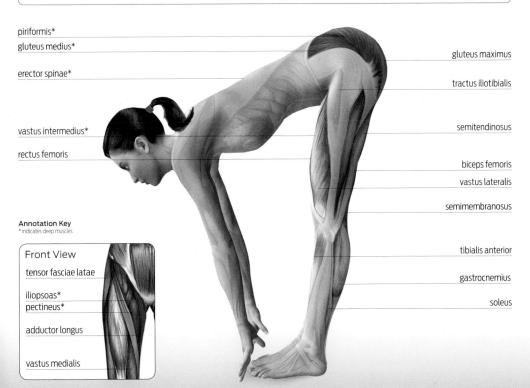

piriformis*

gluteus medius*

erector spinae*

vastus intermedius*

rectus femoris

gluteus maximus

tractus iliotibialis

semitendinosus

biceps femoris

vastus lateralis

semimembranosus

tibialis anterior

gastrocnemius

soleus

Annotation Key
* indicates deep muscles

Front View

tensor fasciae latae

iliopsoas*
pectineus*

adductor longus

vastus medialis

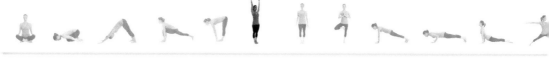

 DVD section 2: Chapter 6

Upward Salute
(Urdhva Hastasana)

Upward Salute is the second pose in the Sun Salutation A series. In the traditional posture, the arms are separated; if your shoulders are more open, you can join your hands together above your head while keeping your arms straight.

1 From Standing Forward Bend (pages 20–21), inhale as you lift your torso up, keeping your back flat as you reach your arms out to your sides, and continue lifting until you are standing with your arms above your head. Your hands should be shoulder-width apart.

2 Straighten your arms, and rotate your shoulders externally open so that the palms of your hands face each other, spreading up through the fingertips.

3 Gaze forward or tilt your head slightly back, and bring your gaze up to your thumbs. Hold for 1 to 5 breaths.

Correct form
· Stretch your arms completely straight from your elbows.
· Soften any tension in your shoulders.

Avoid
· Tensing your shoulders up toward your ears.
· Bending your elbows.

Diary of practice

	Date	No. of Breaths	Comment
Week 1			
Week 2			
Week 3			
Week 4			

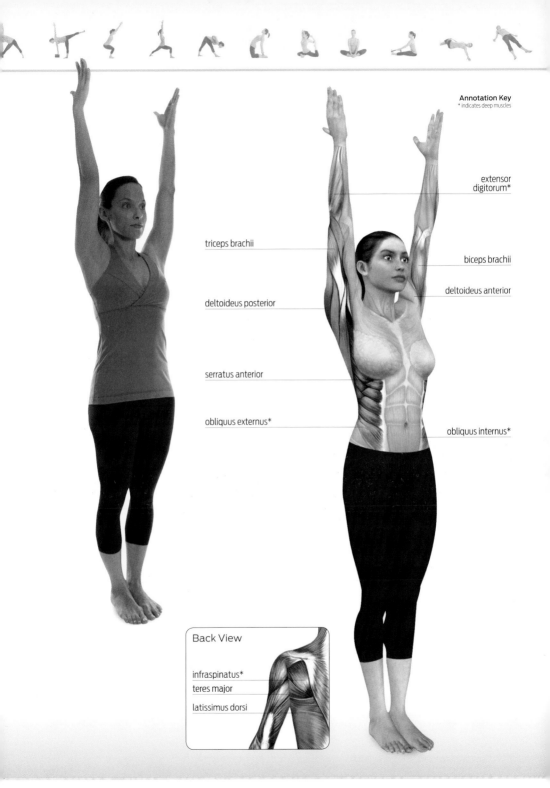

Annotation Key
* indicates deep muscles

extensor
digitorum*

triceps brachii

biceps brachii

deltoideus posterior

deltoideus anterior

serratus anterior

obliquus externus*

obliquus internus*

Back View

infraspinatus*
teres major
latissimus dorsi

Mountain Pose
(Tadasana)

Mountain Pose is the basis for many standing poses. Although this posture may seem simple, it can actually be quite challenging to achieve the correct alignment.

1 From Upward Salute (pages 22–23), exhale as you bring your arms to your sides. Your feet should be together as you stand tall.

2 Breathe in and out as you maintain the pose. Find your balance, keeping your pelvis neutral by drawing the tip of your tailbone down toward your feet as you lift your hip bones upward. Your weight may shift in a circular motion as you balance. Root and rebound, feeling your feet grounded onto the floor as energy radiates from the feet up through the top of your head.

Diary of practice

	Date	No. of Breaths	Comment
Week 1			
Week 2			
Week 3			
Week 4			

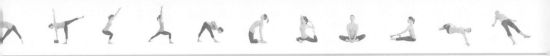

Annotation Key
* indicates deep muscles

Correct form

- Release any tension in the facial area.
- Stand completely straight with shoulders stacked over hips, hips stacked over knees, and knees in line with feet.
- Visualize your pelvis as a bowl of soup—you don't want to spill it forward or backward.
- Stretch your arms straight, with energy reaching out of your fingertips.
- Keep your chin parallel to the floor, and the crown of your head pressing upward.

Avoid

- Arching your lower back.
- Pushing your ribs forward.
- Over-tucking your pelvis.
- Holding your breath.

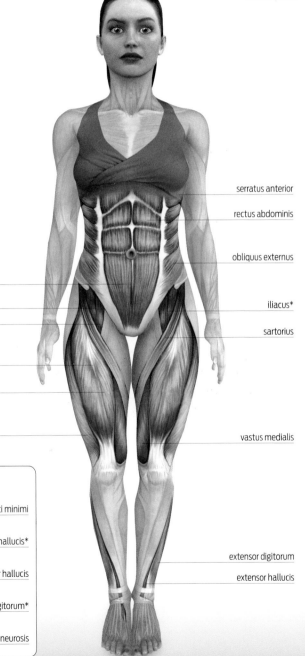

serratus anterior

rectus abdominis

obliquus externus

transversus abdominis*

iliopsoas*

pectineus*

vastus intermedius*

rectus femoris

vastus lateralis

iliacus*

sartorius

vastus medialis

Bottom of Foot

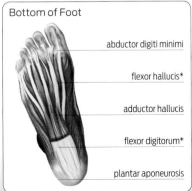

abductor digiti minimi

flexor hallucis*

adductor hallucis

flexor digitorum*

plantar aponeurosis

extensor digitorum

extensor hallucis

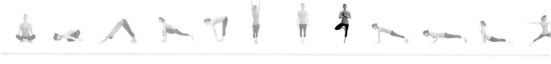

 DVD section 2: Chapter 8

Tree Pose
(Vrksasana)

In Tree Pose, as your standing foot stays strongly rooted to the floor and the top of your head reaches up toward the ceiling, you will feel energy moving down and up at the same time.

1 From Mountain Pose (pages 24–25), bend your right knee, bringing your foot up to your left inner thigh, with toes pointing to the floor.

2 Externally rotate your right thigh, allowing your right knee to point out to the right while keeping your hips level.

3 Continue to open your right hip, rotating your inner thigh clockwise as you draw your tailbone down toward your left heel to neutralize your

pelvis. Press your right foot into your left inner thigh as you draw your left outer hip in for stability.

4 Find your balance, and then join your hands in a prayer position. Hold for 1 to 5 breaths.

5 Release your right foot back down into Mountain Pose (pages 24–25), and repeat the pose on the other leg. Stand in Mountain Pose when finished to begin the Sun Salutation A sequence (page 60).

Diary of practice

	Date	No. of Breaths	Comment
Week 1			
Week 2			
Week 3			
Week 4			

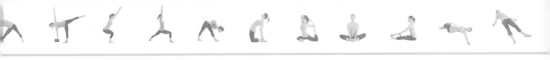

Correct form

- Keep your standing leg in place with the foot facing straight ahead. Ground down through all four corners of this foot to help you balance throughout the exercise.
- If you need help placing your foot at your thigh, grasp the ankle with your hand.
- If you have trouble bringing your foot all the way up to your inner thigh, rest it on the side of your shin instead.
- To assist in balancing, place your heel at your ankle with the ball of the foot on the floor, or lean against a wall.

Avoid

- Resting your foot on the sensitive kneecap area.

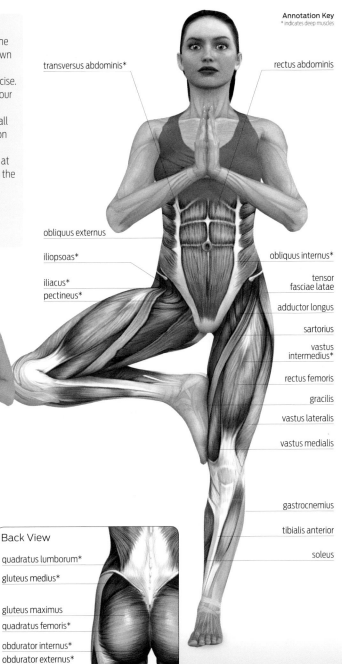

Annotation Key
* indicates deep muscles

transversus abdominis*

rectus abdominis

obliquus externus

iliopsoas*

iliacus*
pectineus*

obliquus internus*

tensor fasciae latae

adductor longus

sartorius

vastus intermedius*

rectus femoris

gracilis

vastus lateralis

vastus medialis

gastrocnemius

tibialis anterior

soleus

Back View

quadratus lumborum*

gluteus medius*

gluteus maximus

quadratus femoris*

obdurator internus*

obdurator externus*

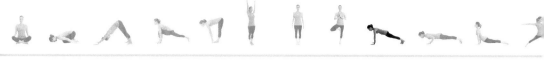

Plank Pose

Plank Pose is part of the traditional Sun Salutation sequence, as well as the vinyasa that you will repeat several times throughout this yoga sequence. This vinyasa consists of Plank Pose, Chaturanga, Upward-Facing Dog, and Downward-Facing Dog. Plank can also be practiced on its own. Challenge yourself by holding it for 30 seconds, 1 minute, or eventually even 2 or 3 minutes.

1 From High Lunge (pages 18–19), place your hands flat on the floor and step your front foot backward to meet your back foot.

2 Inhale, and shift your weight forward so that your shoulders are in line with your wrists. Come onto the balls of your feet with your toes spread out and your heels reaching back. Keep your arms straight and parallel to each other, externally rotating your outer upper arms so that your inner elbows draw forward. As you hold the

pose, soften between your shoulder blades and melt your heart down as you broaden across the collarbones to lift your sternum. Internally rotate your inner thighs, keeping the thighs firm. Lengthen your tailbone down toward your heels. Hold for 1 to 5 breaths.

Correct form
· Make sure that your wrist creases are parallel to the front of the mat.
· Spread your fingers wide, and ground down through every knuckle.
· Use your breath to get you through holding the pose.

Avoid
· Lifting your fingers off the floor.
· Rounding your upper back.

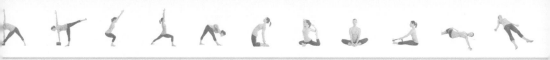

Diary of practice

	Date	No. of Breaths	Comment
Week 1			
Week 2			
Week 3			
Week 4			

Annotation Key
* indicates deep muscles

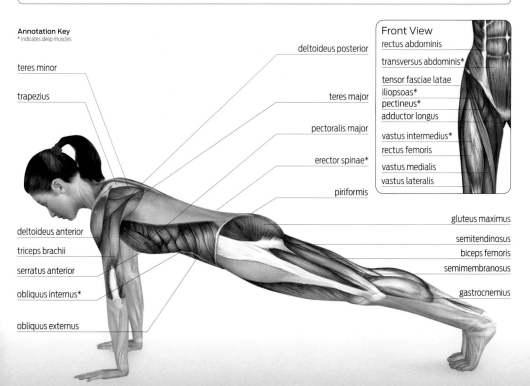

Front View
rectus abdominis
transversus abdominis*
tensor fasciae latae
iliopsoas*
pectineus*
adductor longus
vastus intermedius*
rectus femoris
vastus medialis
vastus lateralis

deltoideus posterior
teres minor
trapezius
teres major
pectoralis major
erector spinae*
piriformis
deltoideus anterior
triceps brachii
serratus anterior
obliquus internus*
obliquus externus
gluteus maximus
semitendinosus
biceps femoris
semimembranosus
gastrocnemius

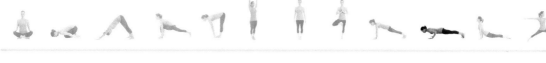

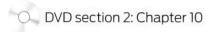

DVD section 2: Chapter 10

Chaturanga
(Chaturanga Dandasana)

Chaturanga, sometimes called Four-Limbed Staff Pose, is practiced in Sun Salutation A and B. It is also part of the vinyasa shown on page 62. Like Plank Pose, Chaturanga challenges your core strength and stability.

1 From Plank Pose (pages 28–29), shift your weight forward toward the tips of your toes. Exhale as you bend your elbows over your wrists and lower yourself down so that your shoulders are in line with your elbows. As you lower, ground your palm and fingers down into the floor. The thumb and index finger have a tendency to want to lift up, so make a special effort to press down between the two.

2 Hold the pose, rotating your inner thighs and drawing your tailbone downward so that you don't sink into your lower back. Lift your thighs away from the floor. Draw your shoulder blades together as you lift the heads of the shoulders away from the floor.

Correct form
· Keep the back of your neck long by gazing slightly beyond the edge of your mat.

Avoid
· Bending your elbows so much that your chest collapses and your shoulders round forward.
· Dropping hips lower than your shoulders.

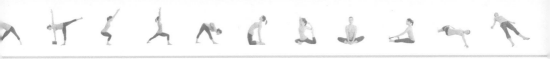

Diary of practice

	Date	No. of Breaths	Comment
Week 1			
Week 2			
Week 3			
Week 4			

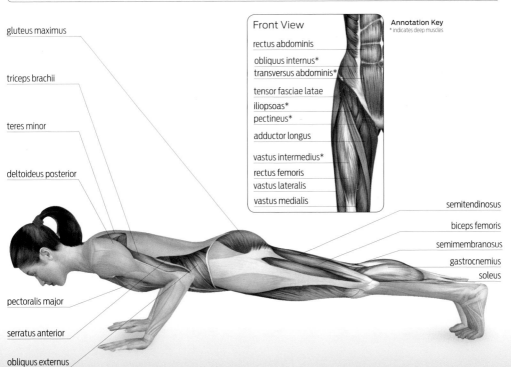

gluteus maximus

triceps brachii

teres minor

deltoideus posterior

pectoralis major

serratus anterior

obliquus externus

Front View

rectus abdominis

obliquus internus*

transversus abdominis*

tensor fasciae latae

iliopsoas*

pectineus*

adductor longus

vastus intermedius*

rectus femoris

vastus lateralis

vastus medialis

Annotation Key
* indicates deep muscles

semitendinosus

biceps femoris

semimembranosus

gastrocnemius

soleus

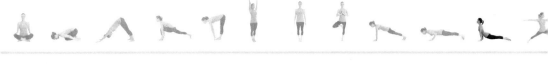

Upward-Facing Dog
(Urdhva Mukha Svanasana)

Upward-Facing Dog is a backbend posture in both of the Sun Salutation sequences. It is also a step in the vinyasa, along with Plank Pose, Chaturanga, and Downward-Facing Dog.

1 From Chaturanga (pages 30–31), inhale and straighten your arms so that your shoulders are directly above your wrists as you flip to the tops of both feet, keeping your thighs and knees off the floor the entire time. Spread your fingers, and ground down. Draw your tailbone down, and lift your pubic bone toward your belly button.

2 To continue the sequence, exhale, lifting your hips up as you simultaneously flip your feet and transition to Downward-Facing Dog. Hold for 1 to 5 breaths.

Correct form
- Keep your wrists parallel to the front edge of your mat, and position your shoulders above your wrists.
- Keep your chin tucked slightly as you lengthen the back of your neck.
- While holding the pose, focus on a comfortable gazing point, such as the spot where wall and ceiling meet.

Avoid
- Resting your thighs on the floor.
- Positioning your hands in front of your shoulders.
- Externally rotating your thighs, as this can compress your lower back.

Diary of practice

	Date	No. of Breaths	Comment
Week 1			
Week 2			
Week 3			
Week 4			

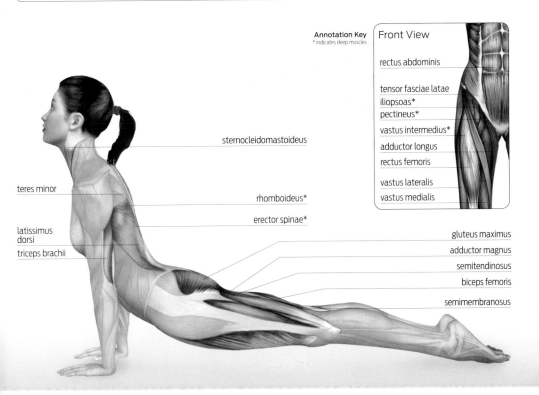

Annotation Key
indicates deep muscles

Front View

rectus abdominis

tensor fasciae latae
iliopsoas*
pectineus*

vastus intermedius*

adductor longus

rectus femoris

vastus lateralis

vastus medialis

sternocleidomastoideus

teres minor

rhomboideus*

erector spinae*

latissimus dorsi

triceps brachii

gluteus maximus

adductor magnus

semitendinosus

biceps femoris

semimembranosus

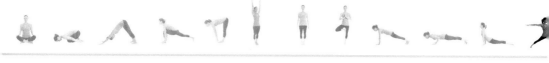

Warrior II
(Virabhadrasana II)

One of the three Warrior poses performed in yoga, Warrior II is often performed earlier in a sequence than Warrior I. Mastering Warrior II will help you build the inner strength and courage of a warrior.

1 From Downward-Facing Dog (pages 16–17), step the right foot forward, to come into High Lunge (pages 18–19).

2 Pivot your left heel down, and turn your foot out 45 degrees. Walk your right foot to the left several inches so that your right heel aligns with the inner arch of your left foot.

3 Keeping your right knee bent, lift your torso so that your shoulders line up over your hips. Keep a slight internal rotation to the back leg to keep the leg neutral. Extend both arms out to the sides, parallel to the floor, with palms facing downward. Continue to bend your right knee so that your thigh is parallel to the floor, externally rotating your right hip to open your thigh. Find a neutral pelvis. Turn your head to the right and gaze past your fingers.

4 Hold for 1 to 5 breaths. Later in the sequence, repeat on the other side.

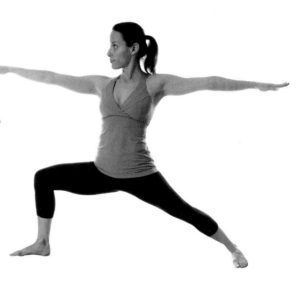

Correct form
- Press your heels into the floor, using your inner-thigh muscles.
- Keep your shoulders directly above your hips.
- When holding the pose, make sure that your front knee is in line with your middle toe.

Avoid
- Arching your lower back.
- Leaning forward over your bent leg.

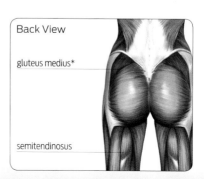

Back View

gluteus medius*

semitendinosus

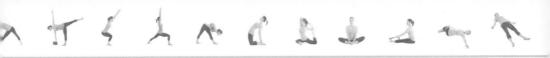

Diary of practice

	Date	No. of Breaths	Comment
Week 1			
Week 2			
Week 3			
Week 4			

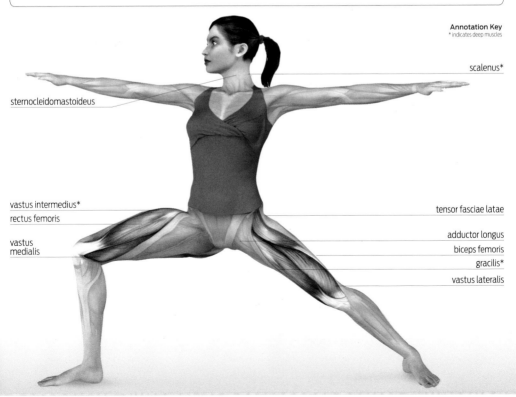

Annotation Key
* indicates deep muscles

scalenus*

sternocleidomastoideus

vastus intermedius*

rectus femoris

vastus medialis

tensor fasciae latae

adductor longus

biceps femoris

gracilis*

vastus lateralis

Extended Triangle with Block
(Utthita Trikonasana)

Extended Triangle Pose encompasses the entire body. It is a hip opener, core strengthener, side bend, twist, and heart opener. This version allows you to use a yoga block, which means less stress on tight hamstrings and hips.

1 From Warrior II (pages 34–35), inhale to straighten your right leg by firming your thigh and lifting your kneecap upward. You may need to shorten your stance by about 6 to 12 inches (15 to 30 cm). Keep your right heel in line with the center of your left foot. Externally rotate your right thigh while keeping your back leg neutral.

2 Keeping both legs straight with firm thighs and your arms extended out to your sides parallel to the floor, exhale and reach your right arm and torso down to the right as you shift your hips to the left, deepening the crease in your right hip.

3 Place your right hand on the block on the outside of your right leg. Extend your left arm straight up, with fingers spread. Inhale as you find length across your collarbones.

4 Exhale, and turn the right side of your torso toward the ceiling.

5 Inhale as you turn your head to gaze up at your left fingertips. Hold for 1 to 5 breaths. Later in the sequence, repeat on the other side.

Correct form
· Bend from your hips, not from your waist.
· Keep your thighs engaged by maintaining a very slight bend in your knees.
· Stand as if you were in between two panes of glass.
· Position the block directly underneath your shoulder.

Avoid
· Straightening your legs so much that your knees lock.
· Crunching the bottom side of your torso while bending.
· Leaning forward.

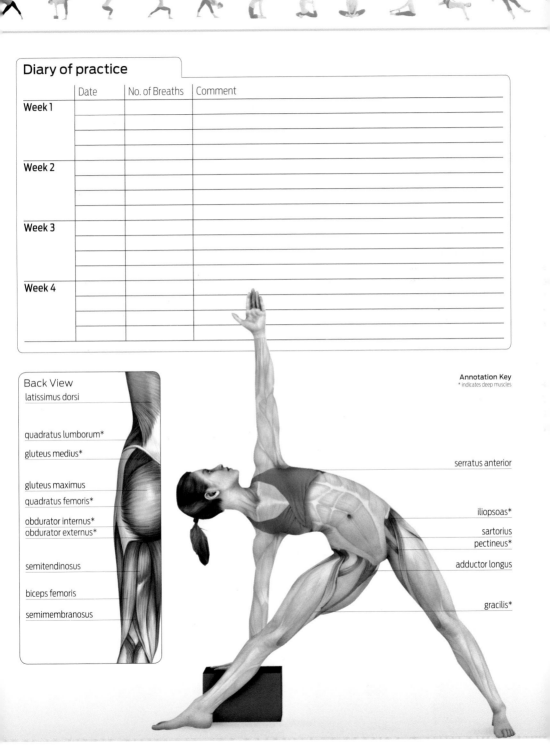

Diary of practice

	Date	No. of Breaths	Comment
Week 1			
Week 2			
Week 3			
Week 4			

Annotation Key
* indicates deep muscles

Back View

latissimus dorsi

quadratus lumborum*

gluteus medius*

gluteus maximus

quadratus femoris*

obdurator internus*
obdurator externus*

semitendinosus

biceps femoris

semimembranosus

serratus anterior

iliopsoas*

sartorius
pectineus*

adductor longus

gracilis*

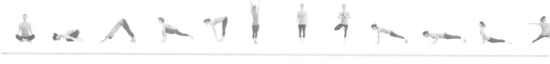

 DVD section 2: Chapter 14

Half Moon with Block
(Ardha Chandrasana)

Half Moon is a hip opener as well as a balancing posture. This version uses a block. With its rectangular shape, the block's sides give you three heights to choose from, depending on how limber you feel during your yoga practice.

1 Stand in Extended Triangle with Block (pages 36–37) with your right palm or fingertips on the block. Keep the alignment you found in Extended Triangle as you turn your gaze downward to your right foot. Bring your left hand onto your hip to help find your balance.

2 Bend your right knee slightly, keeping it extended over your middle toe as you move your block forward about a foot and a half in front of your right small toe. At the same time, shift more weight onto your right leg, and step your left foot in about 12 inches (30 cm).

3 Straighten your right leg, turning the thigh open clockwise while lifting your left leg parallel to the floor to hip height or slightly higher. Keep your left leg in a neutral position, and flex your ankle.

4 Once you have your balance, extend your left arm straight up toward the ceiling, opening up across the front of your chest. Hold for 1 to 5 breaths.

5 To come out of the pose, bring your left hand onto your hip. Bend your right knee, keeping it over your middle toes as you step your left leg back about 3 or 4 feet (1 meter). Straighten your right leg, move the block, and transition back into Extended Triangle, then continue to reverse your steps back into Warrior II.

6 From Warrior II, follow either Transition 1 or Transition 2 (page 63) to end in Downward-Facing Dog. Then, repeat all steps on the left side. After doing both sides, move into Transition 4 (pages 63) to end in Mountain Pose.

Correct form
· Turn your gaze toward the floor, to the side, or up to your raised hand.
· To help activate your lifted leg, imagine that you are pressing your flexed foot into a wall behind you.

Avoid
· Letting your standing foot turn in.
· Allowing the knee of your standing foot to twist out of alignment.

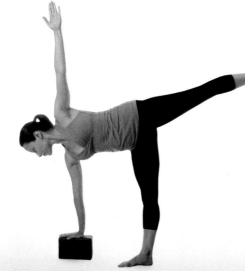

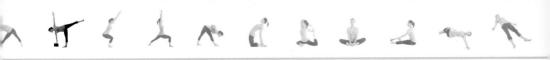

Diary of practice

	Date	No. of Breaths	Comment
Week 1			
Week 2			
Week 3			
Week 4			

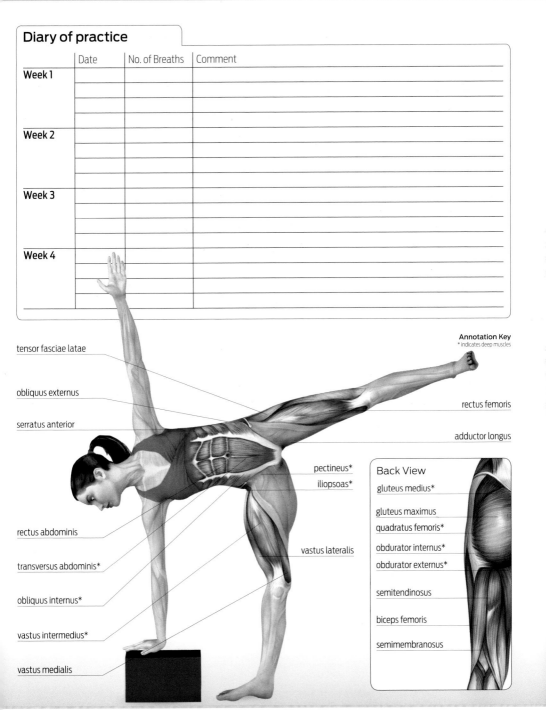

Annotation Key
* indicates deep muscles

tensor fasciae latae

obliquus externus

serratus anterior

rectus femoris

adductor longus

pectineus*
iliopsoas*

rectus abdominis

transversus abdominis*

obliquus internus*

vastus intermedius*

vastus medialis

vastus lateralis

Back View
gluteus medius*
gluteus maximus
quadratus femoris*
obdurator internus*
obdurator externus*
semitendinosus
biceps femoris
semimembranosus

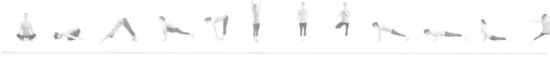

 DVD section 2: Chapter 15

Chair Pose
(Utkatasana)

Chair Pose is a versatile pose, because you can easily control its intensity, bending your knees just a few inches or all the way down so that your hips are in line with your knees. This pose is part of Sun Salutation B.

1 Begin in Mountain Pose (pages 24–25), with your feet together and arms by your sides. Inhale your arms into Upward Salute (pages 22–23), reaching above your head so that your arms are parallel to each other. Rotate your outer upper arms inward and reach up through your fingertips.

2 Exhale, and bend your knees. Both ankles, inner thighs, and knees should be touching. Bring your weight onto your heels, try to shift your hips back, and draw your knees right above your ankles. Hold for 1 to 5 breaths.

3 Straighten your legs and fold forward into Standing Forward Bend to begin the vinyasa, ending in Downward-Facing Dog (pages 16–17).

Correct form
· Find a neutral position by drawing your tailbone down as you roll your inner thighs toward the floor.

Avoid
· Over-tucking your pelvis.
· Over-arching your lower back.
· Letting your feet separate or your knees knock inward.
· Lifting your heels.

Diary of practice

	Date	No. of Breaths	Comment
Week 1			
Week 2			
Week 3			
Week 4			

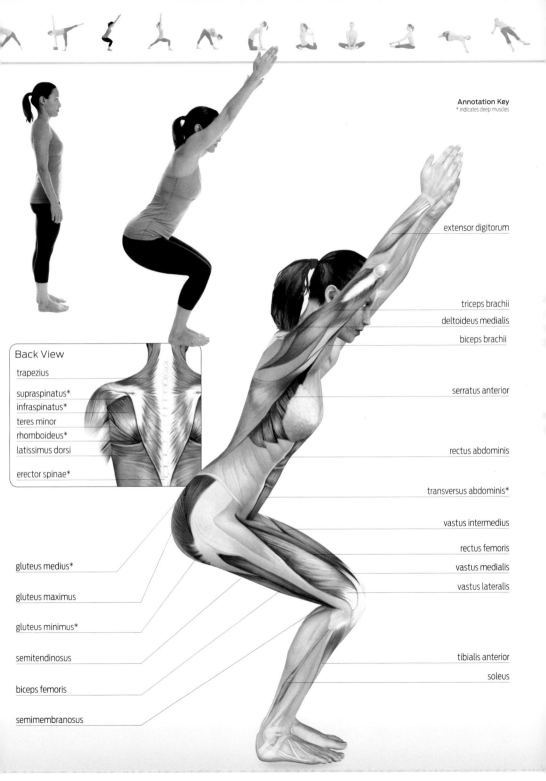

Annotation Key
* indicates deep muscles

extensor digitorum

triceps brachii

deltoideus medialis

biceps brachii

serratus anterior

rectus abdominis

transversus abdominis*

vastus intermedius

rectus femoris

vastus medialis

vastus lateralis

tibialis anterior

soleus

Back View

trapezius

supraspinatus*

infraspinatus*

teres minor

rhomboideus*

latissimus dorsi

erector spinae*

gluteus medius*

gluteus maximus

gluteus minimus*

semitendinosus

biceps femoris

semimembranosus

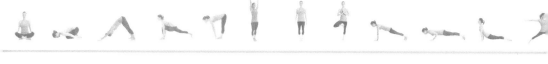

Warrior I
(Virabhadrasana I)

Warrior I requires a mix of fortitude and flexibility. With practice, you will build strength and increase your confidence both on and off the mat.

1 From Downward-Facing Dog (pages 16–17), step your right foot forward into High Lunge (pages 18–19), pivot your left heel down, and angle your left toes to face the upper left corner of your mat. Walk your right foot to the right several inches, so that your feet are in heel-to-heel alignment.

2 Keep your left leg straight and your right knee bent as you inhale, lifting your torso and arms above your head, with your body in a straight line. Externally rotate both arms, palms facing toward each other, and energy up through your fingertips.

3 Hold the pose for 1 to 5 breaths with your shoulders, torso, and hips squared to the front of the mat. Your bent knee should be in line with your middle toe. Aim to bend so that your thigh is parallel to the floor. Press into the outer edge of your left foot and firm your left thigh as you slightly internally rotate the leg.

4 To come out of the pose, place your hands on the floor and lift your left heel back into High Lunge. From High Lunge continue through the entire Sun Salutation B sequence (page 61), including the left side, to end in Mountain Pose (pages 24–25).

Diary of practice

	Date	No. of Breaths	Comment
Week 1			
Week 2			
Week 3			
Week 4			

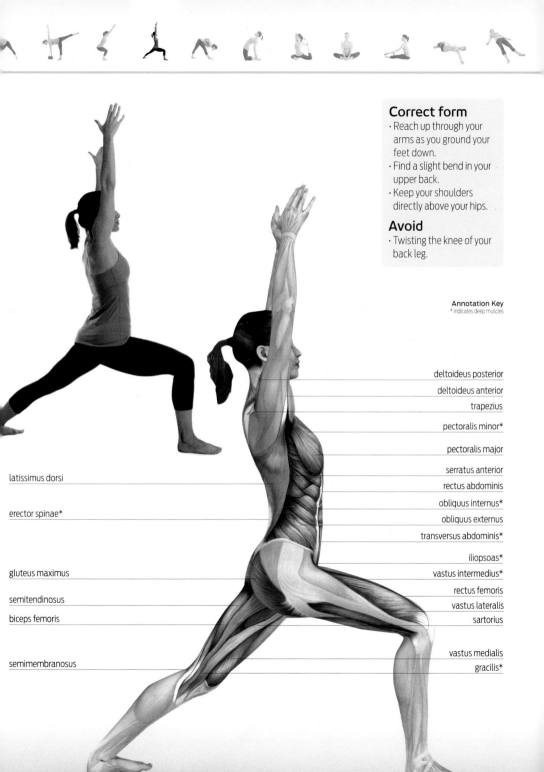

Correct form

· Reach up through your arms as you ground your feet down.
· Find a slight bend in your upper back.
· Keep your shoulders directly above your hips.

Avoid

· Twisting the knee of your back leg.

Annotation Key
* indicates deep muscles

deltoideus posterior

deltoideus anterior

trapezius

pectoralis minor*

pectoralis major

serratus anterior

rectus abdominis

obliquus internus*

obliquus externus

transversus abdominis*

iliopsoas*

vastus intermedius*

rectus femoris

vastus lateralis

sartorius

vastus medialis

gracilis*

latissimus dorsi

erector spinae*

gluteus maximus

semitendinosus

biceps femoris

semimembranosus

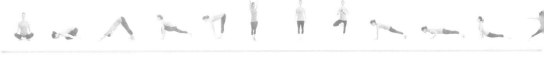

Intense Side Stretch
(Parsvottanasana)

Intense Side Stretch is a forward bend that is calming, while it also provides an intense stretch for your hamstrings—especially beneficial if you like to run.

1 From Mountain Pose (pages 24–25), step your left foot back about 3 feet (1 meter). Turn your toes in about 45 degrees so that they face the upper left corner of your mat. Come into heel-to-heel alignment, squaring your hips to the front of the mat.

2 Extend your arms out parallel to the floor, turn your thumbs down, bend your elbows, and join your hands into a prayer position: begin with the backs of your hands together and the fingers pointing down, and then turn your fingers away from your back and flip your wrists so that your fingers point upward. Press your pinky fingers together, and slowly try to press your hands together.

3 Inhale, broadening across your collar bones, drawing your shoulder blades together and lifting your chest while keeping your hips squared.

4 Ground through the pinky toe edge of your left foot, and press your left thigh back as you exhale to fold forward over your right leg. Lead with your heart and keep your spine elongated. Hold for 1 to 5 breaths.

5 Inhale, draw your shoulders back, and lift your sternum, leading with your heart to come up to standing. Step your left foot forward to meet your right foot in Mountain Pose, and repeat on the other side.

6 Repeat the first nine steps of Sun Salutation A (page 60), ending in Downward-Facing Dog (pages 16–17).

Correct form
· As you square your hips, draw your right hip crease back as you press your right big toe down to counteract that movement.
· If you have tight hamstrings, try widening your stance by walking your right foot closer to the right edge of the mat.

Avoid
· Rounding your back as you fold forward.

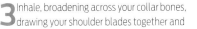
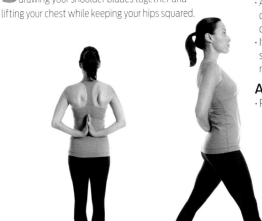
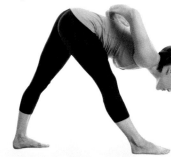

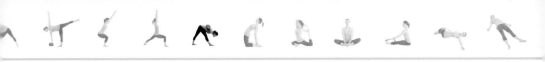

Diary of practice

	Date	No. of Breaths	Comment
Week 1			
Week 2			
Week 3			
Week 4			

gluteus maximus
gluteus medius*
gluteus minimus

semitendinosus

biceps femoris

semimembranosus

gastrocnemius

soleus

Annotation Key
* indicates deep muscles

erector spinae

latissimus dorsi

Front View
tensor fasciae latae
iliopsoas*
pectineus*
vastus intermedius*
adductor longus
rectus femoris
vastus lateralis
vastus medialis

Camel Pose
(Ustrasana)

Camel Pose is a heart-opening backbend that stretches the shoulders and lower back.

1 From Downward-Facing Dog (pages 16–17), come into a kneeling position, with your knees hip-width apart and shins and feet aligned behind them. The tops of your feet should be on the floor, your toes pointing straight back.

2 Bend your elbows, and bring your hands to your lower back, fingers pointing upward. Draw your elbows together, opening your chest. Internally rotate your thighs, and use the heels of your palms to draw your buttocks toward the floor as you lift out of your lower back.

3 Bend from your upper back, and straighten your arms as you reach behind you to grasp your heels. Keep your hips directly above your knees; if your hips shift backward as you reach for your toes, then keep your hands on your lower back. With practice, you will eventually be able to bend back to reach your heels.

4 Broaden across your collarbones and press your shoulder blades in and up to open your chest and shoulders. Allow your head to drop back. Hold for 1 to 5 breaths.

5 To come out of the pose, exhale to lift your head and torso and sit into Child's Pose (pages 14–15), releasing your back. If desired, repeat Camel Pose 2 or 3 times, and then return to Downward-Facing Dog (pages 16–17).

Correct form
· While bending back, keep your thighs perpendicular to the floor.
· If your neck feels stressed when you drop your head back, just keep your head lifted, and gaze forward.

Avoid
· Bending from your hips.
· Arching your lower back.

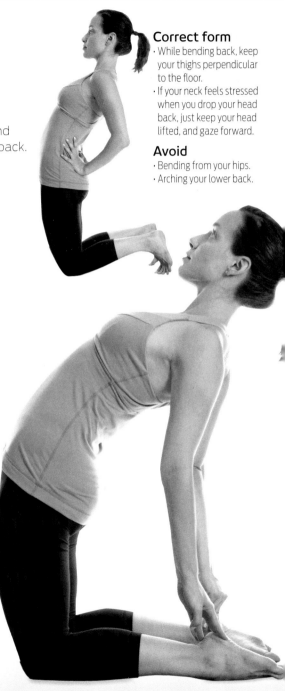

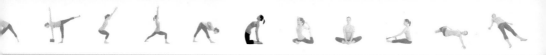

Diary of practice

	Date	No. of Breaths	Comment
Week 1			
Week 2			
Week 3			
Week 4			

sternocleidomastoideus

pectoralis major

rectus abdominis

pectoralis minor*

trapezius

deltoideus posterior
coracobrachialis*

triceps brachii

biceps brachii

gluteus maximus

semitendinosus

biceps femoris

semimembranosus

Annotation Key
* indicates deep muscles

Front View
tensor fasciae latae
iliopsoas*
pectineus*
vastus intermedius*
adductor longus
rectus femoris
vastus lateralis
vastus medialis

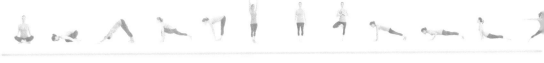

Pigeon Pose
(Eka Pada Rajakapotasana)

Pigeon Pose is a very challenging pose because it demands flexibility in the hips, thighs, spine, and shoulders.

1 From Downward-Facing Dog (pages 16–17), inhale and lift your right leg up behind you.

2 On an exhale, bend your right knee into your chest and then lower your body so that your right knee is on the floor in front of you, foot facing left, right shin and foot on the floor. Draw your right shin slightly forward, and flex your right ankle to keep your knee in alignment.

3 Extend your left leg behind you, with the top of your foot on the floor and toes pointing straight back.

4 Slowly lift your torso upright, bend your left knee, and hold onto your foot with your left hand. Lift up out of the lower back by drawing your tailbone down as you lift your pubic bone toward your frontal hipbones.

5 Bring your foot into the crook of your left elbow before reaching your right arm up, bending the elbow toward the ceiling, and clasping your hands as you continue to square the hips and shoulders. Hold for 1 to 5 breaths.

6 To come out of the pose, straighten your left leg and tuck your left toes under. Place your hands flat onto the floor, straighten your arms and place your right foot onto the floor into High Lunge (pages 18–19). Then step your right leg back into Downward-Facing Dog. Repeat on the other side.

Correct form
· Bend from your thoracic spine.
· Internally rotate your thigh to place your left leg behind you.
· If desired, place padding under your buttocks for support.
· You can place a block or a blanket under your right hip if there is space between your hip and the floor. Support your hips so that you can keep your sacrum level and help square the hips to the front of the mat.

Avoid
· Bending from your lumbar spine.

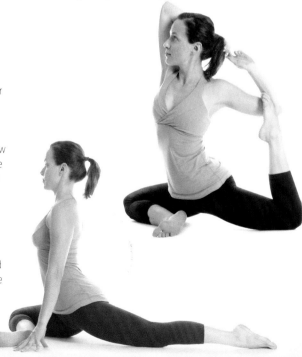

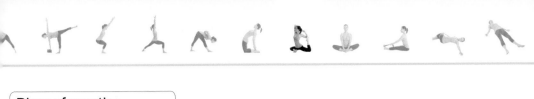

Diary of practice

	Date	No. of Breaths	Comment
Week 1			
Week 2			
Week 3			
Week 4			

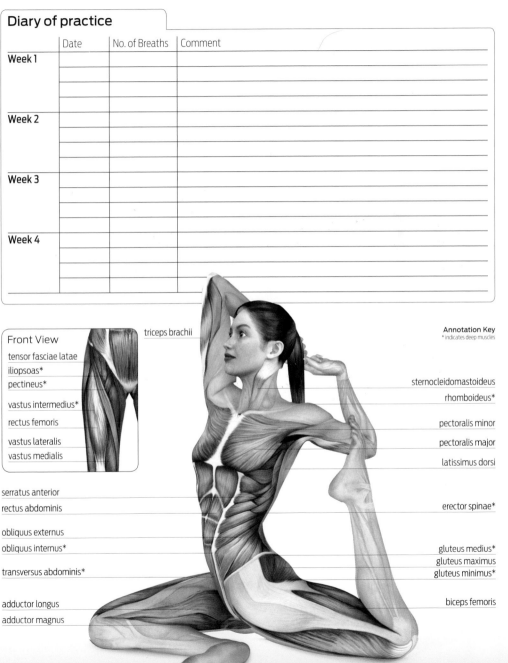

Front View

tensor fasciae latae
iliopsoas*
pectineus*
vastus intermedius*
rectus femoris
vastus lateralis
vastus medialis

triceps brachii

Annotation Key
* indicates deep muscles

sternocleidomastoideus
rhomboideus*
pectoralis minor
pectoralis major
latissimus dorsi

serratus anterior
rectus abdominis

obliquus externus
obliquus internus*

transversus abdominis*

erector spinae*

gluteus medius*
gluteus maximus
gluteus minimus*

adductor longus
adductor magnus

biceps femoris

Bound Angle Pose
(Baddha Konasana)

Beneficial for all levels, Bound Angle Pose is a great hip opener. To execute this pose properly, aim your navel toward your feet—not your head.

1 From Pigeon Pose (48–49), swing your right leg around in front, shifting your weight onto the left hip.

2 Bend both knees and bring the soles of your feet together as you draw your feet in toward your pelvis, keeping your knees apart. Hold your ankles and press the small-toe side of both feet together, "opening" the insides of your feet as if you were opening a book.

3 Inhale as you lengthen your sternum and open your collarbones. Exhale, and fold forward, leading with your heart.

Correct form
· To make the pose feel more restorative, rest your forehead on a block.

Avoid
· Rounding your upper back to fold forward.
· Forcing your knees down.

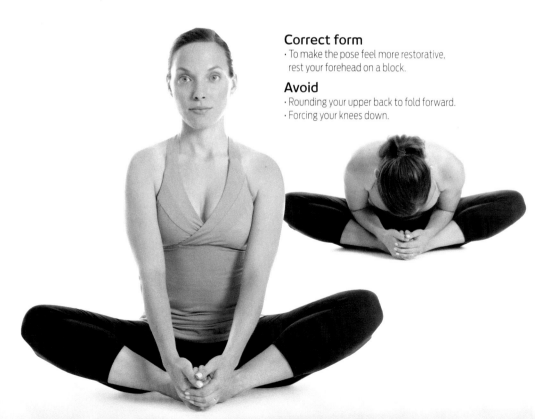

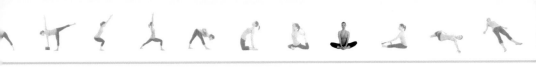

Diary of practice

	Date	No. of Breaths	Comment
Week 1			
Week 2			
Week 3			
Week 4			

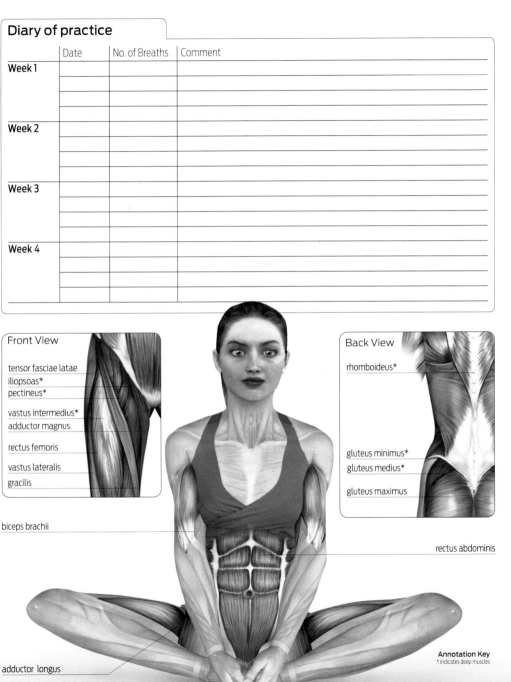

Front View

tensor fasciae latae
iliopsoas*
pectineus*

vastus intermedius*
adductor magnus

rectus femoris

vastus lateralis

gracilis

biceps brachii

Back View

rhomboideus*

gluteus minimus*
gluteus medius*

gluteus maximus

rectus abdominis

adductor longus

Annotation Key
* indicates deep muscles

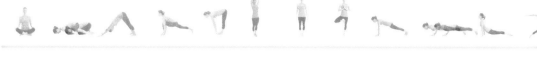

Seated Forward Bend
(Paschimottanasana)

Seated Forward Bend is an introspective posture. It requires you to "surrender," reducing stress and calming the mind. This version uses a yoga strap so that you can keep your spine elongated.

1 From Bound Angle Pose (pages 50–51) lift your knees with your hands until your feet are flat on the floor, and then straighten your legs in front of you with feet flexed. Firm your thighs into the floor.

2 Place your yoga strap under the balls of your feet so that the strap wraps around both feet. Inhale, lengthening your spine, and exhale to fold forward, "walking" your hands forward on the strap.

3 Hinge at your hips and bring your belly toward your thighs. Maintain a slight arch in your lower back as you root your thighs down toward the floor, which will help you to fold more deeply. Inhale to lengthen your spine and exhale to fold farther into your legs.

Correct form
· Lengthen from the base of your spine.
· Lead with your heart.
· Your feet should be straight, as if you were standing in Mountain Pose.

Avoid
· Rounding your upper back.

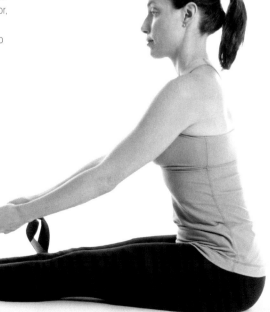

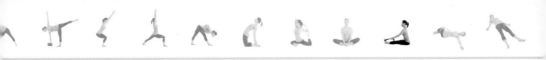

Diary of practice

	Date	No. of Breaths	Comment
Week 1			
Week 2			
Week 3			
Week 4			

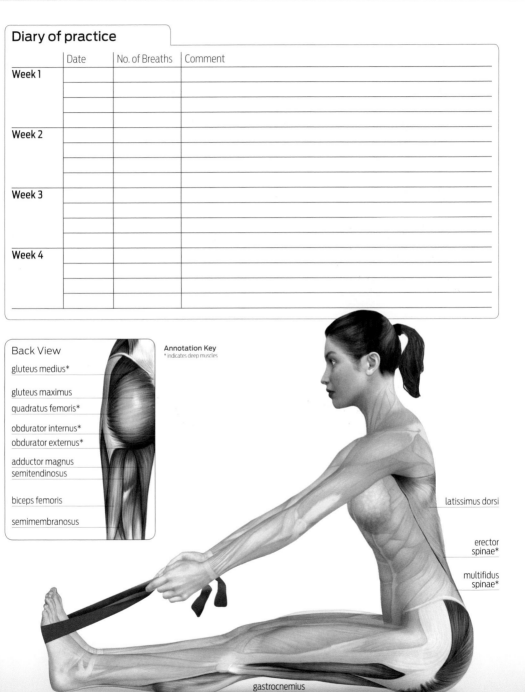

Back View

gluteus medius*

gluteus maximus

quadratus femoris*

obdurator internus*

obdurator externus*

adductor magnus
semitendinosus

biceps femoris

semimembranosus

Annotation Key
* indicates deep muscles

latissimus dorsi

erector
spinae*

multifidus
spinae*

gastrocnemius

Reclining Twist
(Jathara Parivrrti)

Reclining Twist can be performed at any level. It is very relaxing, so you can practice it with your eyes closed before moving into Corpse Pose.

1 Lie on your back. Bend your knees into your chest and extend your arms into a T position with your palms facing downward.

2 Drop both of your knees to the right and hold onto them with your right hand. Twist your upper back around to the left. Turn your head to the left and either close your eyes or gaze toward your left fingertips. Hold for 1 to 5 breaths.

3 Return your knees to center, and then repeat the entire twist in the opposite direction.

Correct form
· Relax into the twist.
· Stack your legs one on top of the other so that the knees, shins, and ankles line up.
· For a deeper twist, lift both shoulders a couple of inches off the floor and then place them back down.

Avoid
· Raising your arms too high if you have shoulder pain.

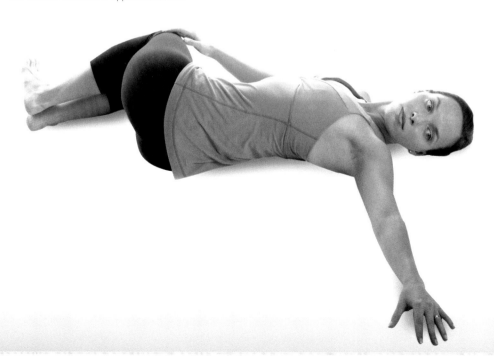

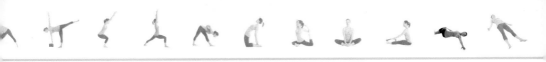

Diary of practice

	Date	No. of Breaths	Comment
Week 1			
Week 2			
Week 3			
Week 4			

obliquus internus*

rectus abdominis

pectoralis major

pectoralis minor*

scalenus*

sternocleidomastoideus

tractus iliotibialis

quadratus lumborum*

obliquus externus

splenius*

levator scapulae*

gluteus maximus

gluteus medius*

serratus anterior

erector spinae*

Annotation Key
* indicates deep muscles

Front View

tensor fasciae latae
iliopsoas*
pectineus*
vastus intermedius*
adductor longus

rectus femoris

vastus lateralis

Corpse Pose
(Savasana)

Corpse Pose, commonly called Savasana, may look easy, but it can be highly challenging. It requires total "surrender" and quieting of the body and mind. Your goal is to let gravity—not your muscles—do the work for you.

1 Lie on your back, and let your arms release outward from your sides far enough from your body for your armpits to have space. Relax your hands and face your palms upward.

2 Let your legs separate to about as wide as your mat so that your lower back starts to release. Allow your legs, feet, and ankles to relax completely. Draw your buttocks down toward your heels to create length in your lower back; to help with this, you can lift your hips slightly and use your hands to draw your buttocks down away from your waist before you completely relax.

3 Let your eyes, jaw, tongue, and throat soften. Release any controlled breath, and begin to breathe quietly. Remain here for 3 to 10 minutes.

4 To transition out of Savasana, inhale and exhale deeply and then start to wiggle your fingers and toes, making small movements to bring awareness back to the rest of the body. Hug both knees into your chest, and then gently roll over onto your right side, taking pressure away from the heart. Pause there for a moment in a fetal position. Slowly press yourself up to sit in Easy Pose (pages 12–13), keeping your eyes closed. Stay there for several breaths (or minutes) before opening your eyes.

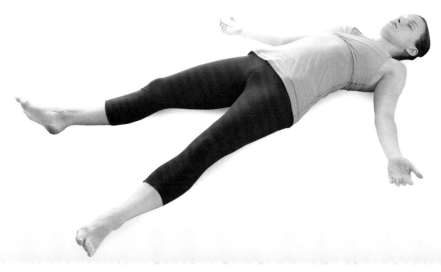

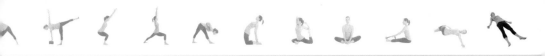

Diary of practice

	Date	No. of Breaths	Comment
Week 1			
Week 2			
Week 3			
Week 4			

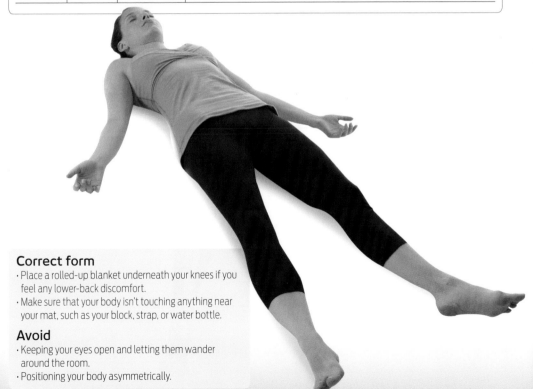

Correct form
· Place a rolled-up blanket underneath your knees if you feel any lower-back discomfort.
· Make sure that your body isn't touching anything near your mat, such as your block, strap, or water bottle.

Avoid
· Keeping your eyes open and letting them wander around the room.
· Positioning your body asymmetrically.

Full-Body Anatomy

Front View

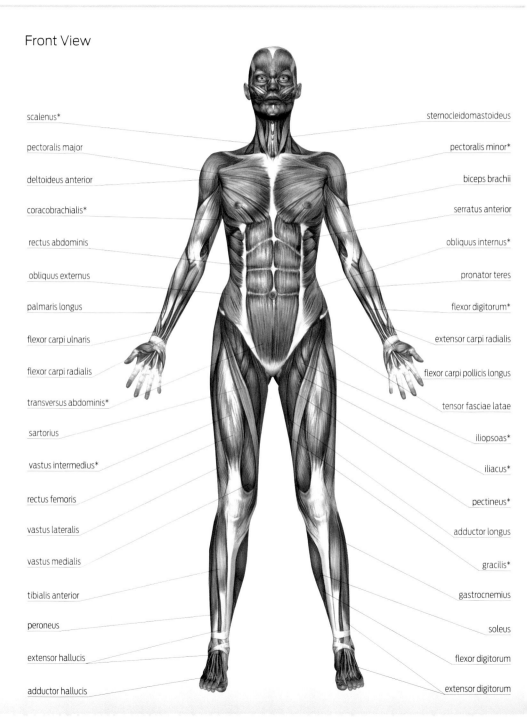

scalenus*

pectoralis major

deltoideus anterior

coracobrachialis*

rectus abdominis

obliquus externus

palmaris longus

flexor carpi ulnaris

flexor carpi radialis

transversus abdominis*

sartorius

vastus intermedius*

rectus femoris

vastus lateralis

vastus medialis

tibialis anterior

peroneus

extensor hallucis

adductor hallucis

sternocleidomastoideus

pectoralis minor*

biceps brachii

serratus anterior

obliquus internus*

pronator teres

flexor digitorum*

extensor carpi radialis

flexor carpi pollicis longus

tensor fasciae latae

iliopsoas*

iliacus*

pectineus*

adductor longus

gracilis*

gastrocnemius

soleus

flexor digitorum

extensor digitorum

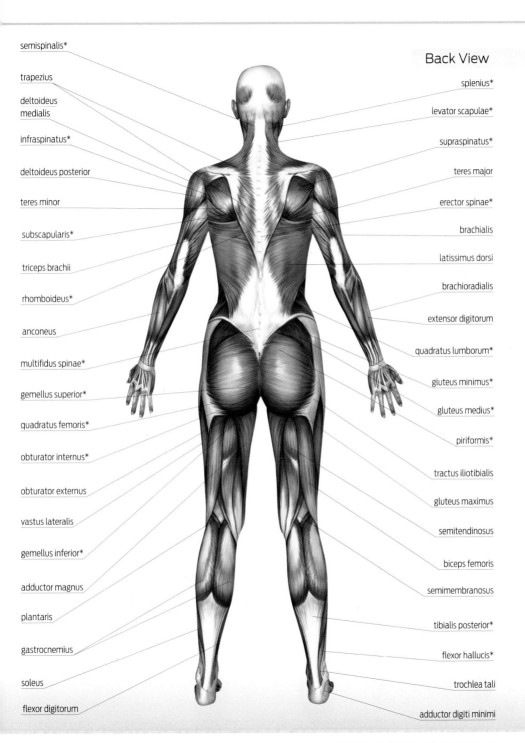

semispinalis*

trapezius

deltoideus
medialis

infraspinatus*

deltoideus posterior

teres minor

subscapularis*

triceps brachii

rhomboideus*

anconeus

multifidus spinae*

gemellus superior*

quadratus femoris*

obturator internus*

obturator externus

vastus lateralis

gemellus inferior*

adductor magnus

plantaris

gastrocnemius

soleus

flexor digitorum

Back View

splenius*

levator scapulae*

supraspinatus*

teres major

erector spinae*

brachialis

latissimus dorsi

brachioradialis

extensor digitorum

quadratus lumborum*

gluteus minimus*

gluteus medius*

piriformis*

tractus iliotibialis

gluteus maximus

semitendinosus

biceps femoris

semimembranosus

tibialis posterior*

flexor hallucis*

trochlea tali

adductor digiti minimi

The Sun Salutations

Sun Salutation A

Sun Salutation A can be performed 2 to 5 times to build heat.

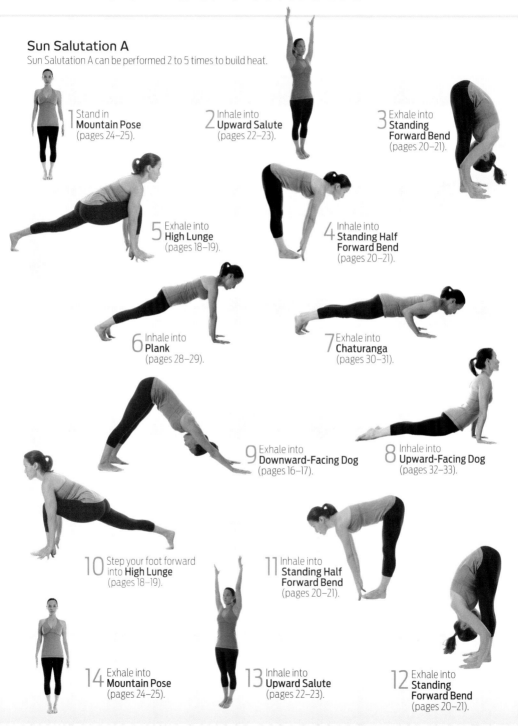

1 Stand in **Mountain Pose** (pages 24–25).

2 Inhale into **Upward Salute** (pages 22–23).

3 Exhale into **Standing Forward Bend** (pages 20–21).

4 Inhale into **Standing Half Forward Bend** (pages 20–21).

5 Exhale into **High Lunge** (pages 18–19).

6 Inhale into **Plank** (pages 28–29).

7 Exhale into **Chaturanga** (pages 30–31).

8 Inhale into **Upward-Facing Dog** (pages 32–33).

9 Exhale into **Downward-Facing Dog** (pages 16–17).

10 Step your foot forward into **High Lunge** (pages 18–19).

11 Inhale into **Standing Half Forward Bend** (pages 20–21).

12 Exhale into **Standing Forward Bend** (pages 20–21).

13 Inhale into **Upward Salute** (pages 22–23).

14 Exhale into **Mountain Pose** (pages 24–25).

Sun Salutation B

Sun Salutation B can be performed 2 to 5 times to build heat.

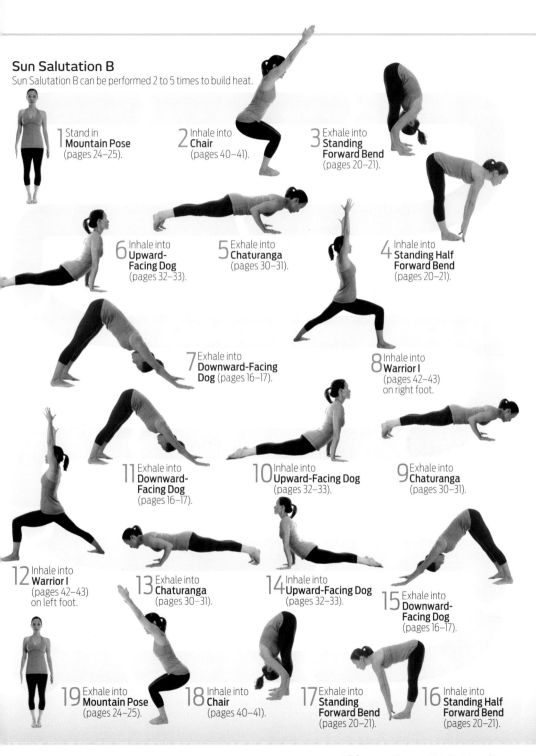

1 Stand in **Mountain Pose** (pages 24–25).

2 Inhale into **Chair** (pages 40–41).

3 Exhale into **Standing Forward Bend** (pages 20–21).

4 Inhale into **Standing Half Forward Bend** (pages 20–21).

5 Exhale into **Chaturanga** (pages 30–31).

6 Inhale into **Upward-Facing Dog** (pages 32–33).

7 Exhale into **Downward-Facing Dog** (pages 16–17).

8 Inhale into **Warrior I** (pages 42–43) on right foot.

9 Exhale into **Chaturanga** (pages 30–31).

10 Inhale into **Upward-Facing Dog** (pages 32–33).

11 Exhale into **Downward-Facing Dog** (pages 16–17).

12 Inhale into **Warrior I** (pages 42–43) on left foot.

13 Exhale into **Chaturanga** (pages 30–31).

14 Inhale into **Upward-Facing Dog** (pages 32–33).

15 Exhale into **Downward-Facing Dog** (pages 16–17).

16 Inhale into **Standing Half Forward Bend** (pages 20–21).

17 Exhale into **Standing Forward Bend** (pages 20–21).

18 Inhale into **Chair** (pages 40–41).

19 Exhale into **Mountain Pose** (pages 24–25).

Vinyasa & Other Transitions

Vinyasa

The vinyasa is a sequence that you will repeat several times during your yoga practice to transition between sustained poses performed to the left or the right. As you become more adept, you will begin to smoothly flow through these movements.

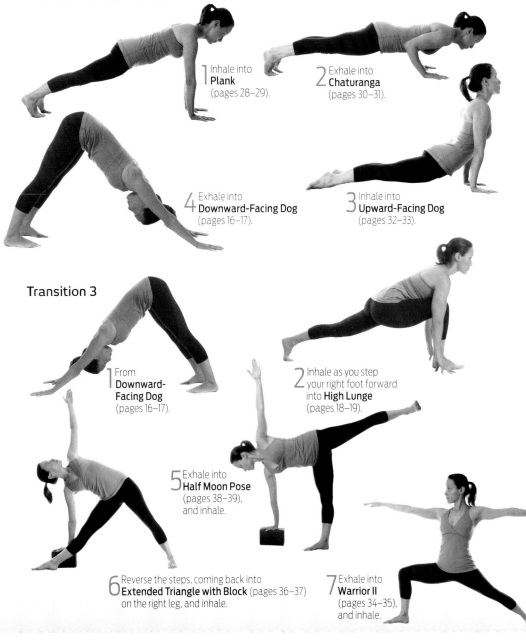

1 Inhale into **Plank** (pages 28–29).

2 Exhale into **Chaturanga** (pages 30–31).

3 Inhale into **Upward-Facing Dog** (pages 32–33).

4 Exhale into **Downward-Facing Dog** (pages 16–17).

Transition 3

1 From **Downward-Facing Dog** (pages 16–17).

2 Inhale as you step your right foot forward into **High Lunge** (pages 18–19).

5 Exhale into **Half Moon Pose** (pages 38–39), and inhale.

6 Reverse the steps, coming back into **Extended Triangle with Block** (pages 36–37) on the right leg, and inhale.

7 Exhale into **Warrior II** (pages 34–35), and inhale.

Other important transitions

You will repeat these sequences throughout your yoga practice.

Transition 1
· Inhale from **Warrior II** (pages 34–35).
· Move into **Plank** (pages 28–29).
· Exhale to **Downward-Facing Dog** (pages 16–17).

Transition 2
· From **Warrior II** (pages 34–35), inhale to begin the **vinyasa** (see opposite), ending in **Downward-Facing Dog** (pages 16–17).

Transition 3 (pictured below)
· From **Downward-Facing Dog** (pages 16–17), inhale as you step your right foot forward into **High Lunge** (pages 18–19).
· Pivot your left heel down, exhale and come into **Warrior II** (pages 34–35), and inhale.
· Exhale into **Extended Triangle with Block** (pages 36–37) on the right leg, and inhale.

· Exhale into **Half Moon Pose with Block** (pages 38–39), and inhale.
· Reverse the steps, coming back into **Extended Triangle with Block** (pages 36–37) on the right leg, and inhale.
· Exhale into **Warrior II** (pages 34–35), and inhale.
· Exhale into **High Lunge** (pages 18–19), and inhale.
· Exhale to **Downward-Facing Dog** (pages 16–17).

Transition 4
· From **Downward-Facing Dog** (pages 16–17) step into **High Lunge** (pages 18–19), then come to the front of your mat.
· Inhale, and lengthen the spine into **Standing Half Forward Bend** (pages 20–21).
· Exhale to **Standing Forward Bend** (pages 20–21).
· Inhale to **Upward Salute** (pages 22–23).
· Exhale to **Mountain Pose** (pages 24–25).

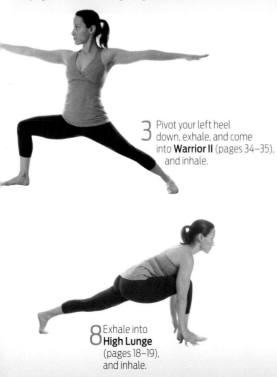

3 Pivot your left heel down, exhale, and come into **Warrior II** (pages 34–35), and inhale.

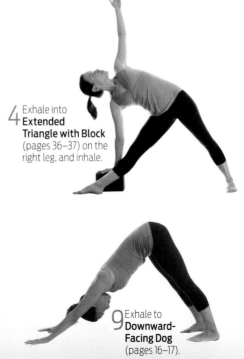

4 Exhale into **Extended Triangle with Block** (pages 36–37) on the right leg, and inhale.

8 Exhale into **High Lunge** (pages 18–19), and inhale.

9 Exhale to **Downward-Facing Dog** (pages 16–17).

About the Author

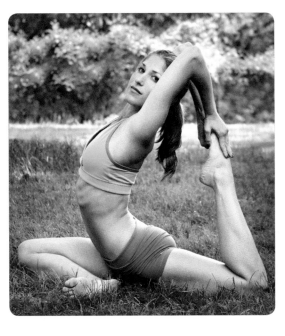

Goldie Karpel Oren began ballet training at the age of three and continued training through high school. During high school she performed with Dances Patrelle in New York as well as Ballet Rox in Boston. She received a B.A from Johns Hopkins University, Baltimore, in 2006, with a major in creative writing. After graduating from college she was a soloist with the Atlantic City Ballet. In spring 2008, Goldie developed an injury that forced her to stop dancing but led her to yoga, which became another passion. Goldie studied yoga and became RYT certified. She now teaches yoga at several studios and works individually with private clients in their homes in New York City. This is Goldie's first published work.

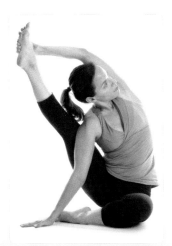

Yoga model Lana Russo is a 500-hour registered yoga teacher with the Yoga Alliance. She earned her training through the Long Island Yoga School in New York and is currently a teacher trainer there, helping others on their journey toward teaching yoga. Lana teaches at many studios throughout the Long Island area and is a current yoga ambassador for Lululemon Athletica. As a former ballet dancer, she enjoys the flow of vinyasa yoga and loves to help bring students to their own personal edge. In her spare time, she enjoys being with her husband and daughter.

ANATOMY ᴼꜰ FITNESS™

Core

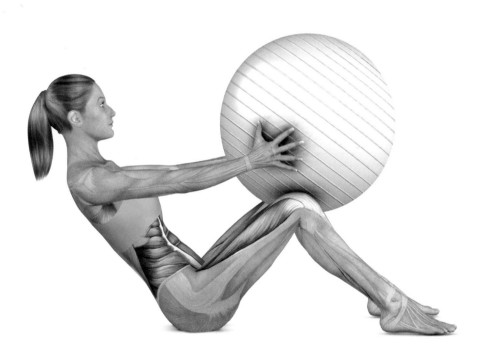

Created by Moseley Road Inc.
Editorial director: Lisa Purcell
Art director: Brian MacMullen
Cover and internals designer: Sam Grimmer
Photographer: Jonathan Conklin Photography, Inc.
Author: Hollis Lance Liebman
Models: Hollis Lance Liebman, Cori D. Cohen
Illustrator: Hector Aiza/3DLabz
Inset illustrations: Linda Bucklin/Shutterstock.com,
page 69 FXQuadro/Shutterstock.com,
page 70 Christopher Edwin Nuzzaco/Shutterstock.com,
page 71 Darrin Henry/Shutterstock.com
Prepress: Graphic Print Group

Contents

Understanding Your Core

This powerful group of muscles seems to have taken center stage in the world of fitness—and rightfully so.

Today's fitness enthusiasts invoke the term *core* so often that it can be hard to tell what the word really means. It is used in myriad ways—by everyone from the new mother wanting to firm her midsection to the weekend tennis warrior seeking more power in his backhand swing or the sedentary executive just looking to get through the day without lower-back pain. And for anyone who wants improved posture or simply to look slimmer and fitter, the idea of "working the core" holds great currency.

What is the core?

The core comprises a system of muscles in the lower trunk area including the lower back, abdomen, and hips. These muscles work together to provide support and mobility, and it is in them that all bodily movement, in every conceivable direction, originates.

The major core muscles include the abdominals, the spinal extensors, and the hip flexors and extensors. The abdominal muscles, or the "abs," consist of the rectus abdominis, transversus abdominis, and the internal and external obliques. The rectus abdominis, commonly called the "six-pack," is responsible for maintaining spine stability as well as shortening the distance between your torso and hips. The transversus abdominis provides thoracic and pelvic stability. Both the internal and external obliques are responsible for your ability to bend from side to side and rotate your torso. The Christmas tree-shaped erector spinae is actually a group of muscles and tendons that stretches from the lumbar to the cervical spine. The erector spinae is responsible for stabilization as well as movement of your spine. The hip flexors (iliopsoas, iliacus, rectus femoris, sartorius, tensor fasciae latae, pectineus, adductor longus, adductor brevis, and gracilis) and hip extensors (gluteus maximus, biceps femoris, semitendinosus, and semimembranosus) act as the basement of this muscular powerhouse, supporting movement and allowing you to flex and extend your hips.

A strong core is paramount to keeping the body functionally sound and operational. Many quick-fix diets, pieces of exercise equipment, and even surgeries promise a sleeker, better-looking abdominal area, but it is through core training that focuses on strength and flexibility—coupled with a healthy diet—that real, long-lasting results can come about.

Everyday benefits

Aside from the obvious aesthetic benefits of maintaining a lean and tight core, there are real-world pluses. Imagine easing back pain, standing up straighter (and in the process, looking taller), and being able to move heavy objects without stress or strain. Performing everyday movements becomes easier, even with age. Core training is an insurance policy for keeping the body functional.

Maintaining a strong core will lend optimal support to ancillary (assisting) muscles. In fact, the core is so central to your body's movement that it is called upon whenever any muscle in the body is used. The core constantly assists other muscle groups, acting as the fulcrum for all motion. For example, lifting an object overhead mainly recruits your deltoids and triceps, but your core muscles also work to both support and balance you, keeping your torso steady as you lift. If your core were not present and firing, it would make proper trunk alignment nearly impossible. That kind of motion, unassisted by the core, would be both much more difficult and potentially dangerous due to spinal compression.

The core is the only muscle system in the body that we train for compactness, rather than for volume as we tend to do with chest muscles. As we train our cores, the ultimate goal is not only to have a sleek, great-looking midsection, but also to attain a functionally sound core that can rotate, contract, and support us in all areas of life.

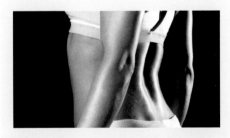

Stronger core = stronger body

Our widespread dependence on artificial support, such as chair backings that shoulder the work of sitting up straight for us, has left many of us soft around the middle. Imagine all of those hours spent slouching, without challenging the core, until upon rising the back feels strained to the point where pain prevails. If you have a sedentary job, you are likely to benefit greatly from challenging your core.

Getting Fit at Home

Core training doesn't have to be expensive. Anyone can follow an effective workout in the privacy of home.

Don't think that you need a huge, intimidating health club with all the latest equipment and extras in order to cultivate an attention-grabbing physique. In truth, some of the fittest bodies have been sculpted in not only less-than-desirable gyms but even in the home with some basic equipment, the desire to improve, and a plan. In fact, a targeted fitness plan performed at home can prove superior to a schedule at a commercial health club that includes a daunting array of high-tech machinery and filled-up classes. At home, you can focus without distractions and at your own pace, experimenting as you see fit in order to keep your workouts interesting.

Home-gym equipment

You need very little equipment for effective at-home core training—your own body weight is your best asset, providing resistance. To add variety to your workout, take advantage of objects around the house: chairs can be used for dips and push-ups, while steps can accommodate lunges. Broomsticks come in handy for balancing exercises and twisting movements. If you don't have a mat, a large, thick towel or carpeting will provide light cushioning and prevent you from sliding on the floor.

Your workout wardrobe

Think comfort, utility, and yes, style when deciding what to wear for your workout. Invest in sneakers or trainers with good cushioning and support; your feet are your foundation.

Dress for breathability, insulation, and functional comfort, choosing garments that allow you to move freely. This doesn't mean that you should throw on shapeless T-shirts or baggy sweatpants; form-fitting shorts and tops move with your natural musculature rather than restricting it. Exercise in front of a mirror whenever possible, too. At the start of your workout plan, you may not like how you look in

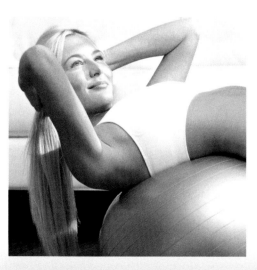

body-hugging garments, but as you stick to your plan, you'll see the changes to your shape even more clearly. Now *that's* motivation!

A time and place for fitness

Effective exercise begins with setting aside a time and a place. This is your chance to give back to your body and maintain the machine that is you. To get the most out of your effort, the location should be free of distractions and allow for clear focus on the task at hand. Elements like music, room temperature, and lighting all have an effect on ensuring the best possible workout. A great thing about working out at home is that you can keep these elements personalized to your own taste.

Make sure that your workout surface is comfortable. If you are exercising on a mat, roll it out properly, ensuring that it is flat, with no loose ends curling upward.

Leave plenty of space around the mat. It is important that you can freely elongate your muscles; incomplete extensions can lead to incomplete muscular development. A full range of motion is vital to your progress.

Now that you are set to begin your workout, you must be present. This may seem like a no-brainer at first, but in today's ultra-fast-paced world, it is easy to become distracted by what you think you may be missing while working out. Try to leave all of your concerns outside your workout space; the world will still exist in all its complexity once your session is over.

For many, making time and space to take care of the body is the hardest part; simply getting ready to exercise, whether this involves going to the gym or setting up a mat at home, takes discipline, time management, and commitment. Now, make the most of it by bettering you.

Fitness balls
A low-tech extra like the antiburst fitness ball shown in several of the following exercises will add another dimension to your at-home routine. This heavy-duty inflatable ball—known by many names, including Swiss ball, exercise ball, body ball, and balance ball—was originally developed for use by physical therapy patients, but it is now standard equipment in commercial and home gyms everywhere. Working on a fitness ball, which ranges in size from 14 to 34 inches (35–85 cm), calls for you to constantly adjust your balance, which forces the engagement of many more muscles, especially those of your core. You can perform both core-stabilizing and core-strengthening exercises on a fitness ball.

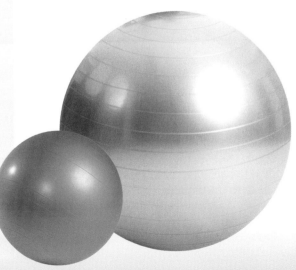

Core Training Basics

Most weight-resistance programs target specific muscle groups, but core training is about treating the body as a unified whole. Although you may feel some of the exercises in this book in one region of your body more strongly than in others, these core workouts are designed to improve muscular function, strengthening, and stabilization throughout your entire body.

You draw upon your core muscles every single day. Although rarely in daily life will you find yourself contracting your biceps or extending your arms to full lockout from your chest as if you're doing a bench press, it's not uncommon to lift an object off the ground and rotate your trunk in order to put it down. This movement is accomplished through reliance on not one isolated muscle, but rather on a group of muscles, including the core, working together.

Breathing, speed, and form are key when working the core. With a firm command of these three elements, you can develop your core muscles efficiently and effectively. Endless repetitions are neither necessary nor advisable; you need only carry out a few calculated sets to achieve a deep muscular burn.

Your breathing pace should be natural and steady. Couple a deep inhale with the negative, or stretching, of the muscle. Think of the inhalation as pulling back the arrow on a bow before launch, and follow it with a deep exhale on the positive, or extended, portion of the movement, as if you were releasing the arrow. Aim for a slow or controlled negative followed by an explosive positive and a slight hold at the peak contraction or finished position. Neither rush through your reps nor greatly slow them; instead, adopt a natural pace that you can sustain throughout the set.

For best results, give your all during each and every rep performed. That guy who claims that he can do a thousand sit-ups would in reality be lucky to complete a hundred that truly work his core, because the neck and lower back—not to mention speed and momentum—are usually called into play when so many repetitions are involved. For best results, less is more: aim to lengthen the muscle, then contract and squeeze. Place the tension on the core muscles at hand without calling in recruits.

Warming up

The following pages include two warm-up stretches followed by both core-stabilizing and core-strengthening exercises. Warm-ups are essential components of a successful fitness regime. You should perform two kinds: cardiovascular exercises and stretches. Jumping rope, boxing, running, cycling—any sustained exertion that gets your heart pumping—will get blood and oxygen moving through your body. Stretches will improve your flexibility, which in turn decreases your risk of injury.

Core stability

Core-stabilizing exercises help to support your core during motion. To stabilize is to both secure your spine and work your visible abdominal muscles. During the execution of a core-stabilizing exercise, your spine should remain in a neutral position without any movement.

Stability exercises focus on improving your core functionality over defining your abdominal musculature.

Core strength

Core-strengthening exercises work the core directly, building strength and endurance as well as muscles. These are the moves that can give you the "six-pack" abs look, in which each segment of the rectus abdominis is highly defined.

Core-strengthening exercises generally target the rectus abdominis, transversus abdominis, and obliques. In the process, the muscles of the midsection become more compact.

Nutrition for core training

When we train our cores, we are aiming for a physique that is both low in visible body fat and high in lean muscle tissue—a physique most definitely achievable. You can maintain a fit core over the long term by carrying out a solid day-to-day plan that combines stretching and strengthening exercises with sound food choices.

For best results, you must fuel properly. The old adage that you are what you eat applies quite literally to the physique. Almost anyone can achieve a "thin" or even "skinny" state by severely limiting food intake, but relying on a drastic reduction of calories often comes at the expense of precious muscle tissue. And a starvation diet usually results in a rebound effect, with the overzealous dieter soon gaining back all of the lost weight and then some.

When it comes to fat loss, the most common mistake lies in overtraining, and in the process breaking the body down to the point of lethargy and exhaustion, while also failing to eat enough to power the body. Too many of us skip breakfast or depend on a last-minute stimulant like coffee—which may fuel us through a few hours—but burnout is inevitable. For optimal results, consume small, frequent meals throughout the day in order to keep your body energized, sparing muscle and instead utilizing stored fat as fuel.

The kinds of food that make up an ideal diet can be divided into three groups: proteins, which help to build muscle mass; fats, which are good for joint lubrication, maintaining body temperature, and promoting healthy cell function in our hair and skin; and carbohydrates, which provide energy.

Half-Kneeling Rotation

Warming up is essential before any workout. The following two exercises will improve your flexibility. Half-Kneeling Rotation is a warm-up stretch that increases your spinal mobility, improves your posture, and enhances your core rotation.

1 Kneel on one leg with your right leg bent at 90 degrees in front of you, foot on the floor. Your hands should be beside your head and your elbows should be flared outward.

2 Keeping your back straight, rotate your left shoulder toward your right knee. Hold for 10 seconds, and then repeat on the other side. Work up to 10 repetitions per side.

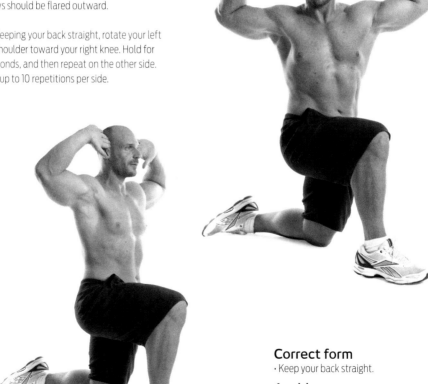

Correct form
· Keep your back straight.

Avoid
· Overextension.

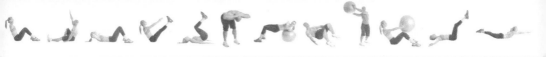

Diary of practice

	Date	Repetitions	Comment
Week 1			
Week 2			
Week 3			
Week 4			

 DVD section 2: Chapter 2

Supine Lower-Back Stretch

Supine Lower-Back Stretch is an excellent warm-up that stretches your lower-back and gluteal muscles.

1 Lie on your back, with legs bent and hands clasped around your knees.

2 Slowly pull your knees toward your chest until you feel a stretch in your lower back.

3 Hold for 30 seconds, relax, and repeat for an additional 30 seconds.

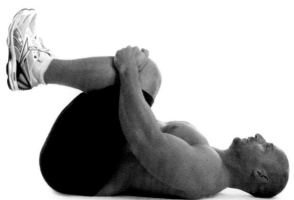

Correct form
· Keep your knees and feet together.

Avoid
· Raising your head off the floor.

Plank

Plank is an isometric, or contracted, core-stabilizing exercise, designed to work your entire core. It is performed everywhere from yoga and Pilates studios to hard-core gyms for a good reason: it is a reliable way to build endurance in your abs and back, as well as the stabilizer muscles.

1 Begin on an exercise mat on your hands and knees in a facedown position.

2 Plant your forearms on the floor, parallel to each other.

3 Raise your knees off the floor and lengthen your legs until they are in line with your arms. Remain suspended in Plank for 30 seconds, building up to 2 minutes.

Correct form
· Keep your abdominal muscles tight.
· Keep your body in a straight line.

Avoid
· Bridging too high, which can take stress off working muscles.

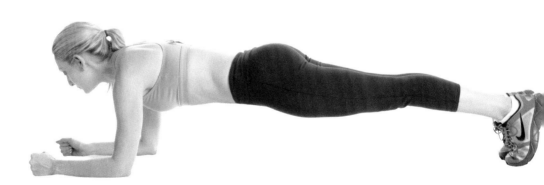

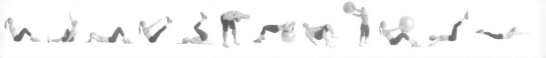

Diary of practice

	Date	Time held	Comment
Week 1			
Week 2			
Week 3			
Week 4			

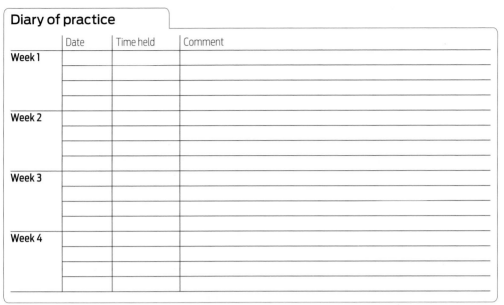

Annotation Key
* indicates deep muscles

Front View

obliquus externus
rectus abdominis
obliquus internus*
transversus abdominis*

adductor longus

rectus femoris

vastus medialis

Back View

semitendinosus

biceps femoris

semimembranosus

gastrocnemius

soleus

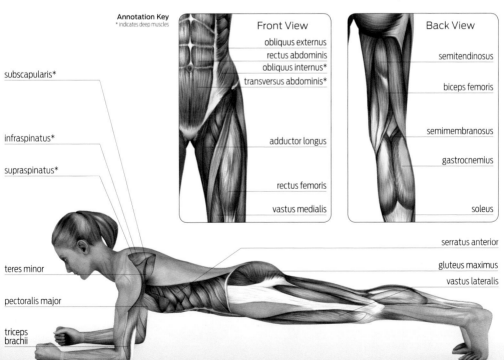

subscapularis*

infraspinatus*

supraspinatus*

teres minor

pectoralis major

triceps brachii

serratus anterior

gluteus maximus

vastus lateralis

Plank-Up

Plank-Up is an advanced core-stabilizing exercise that expands upon the basic Plank exercise. Try to maintain a steady rhythm.

1 Begin on your hands and knees in a facedown position. Plant your forearms on the floor parallel to each other.

2 Raise your knees off the floor and lengthen your legs until they are in line with your arms.

3 Lift up with your right arm until it is fully extended, and then straighten your left arm until you are balanced on both arms in a completed push-up position.

4 Reverse one arm at a time, lowering from the planted hand to forearm until back in the initial plank position. Begin with 10 complete repetitions and work up to 2 sets of 15.

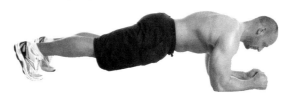

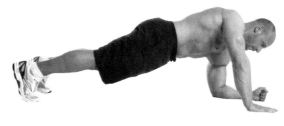

Correct form
· Plant each hand, rather than using momentum, which places too much stress on the joints.
· Keep your abs tucked tightly during the movement.

Avoid
· Crashing down suddenly. Instead, use a steady 4-count motion: 2 up for both arms, then 2 down.

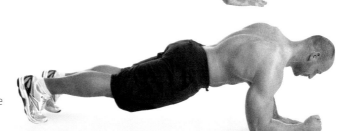

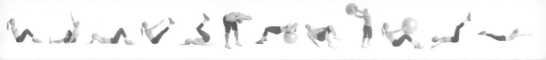

Diary of practice

	Date	Repetitions	Comment
Week 1			
Week 2			
Week 3			
Week 4			

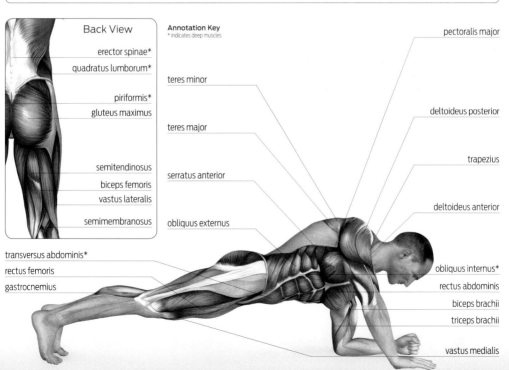

Back View

erector spinae*

quadratus lumborum*

piriformis*

gluteus maximus

semitendinosus

biceps femoris

vastus lateralis

semimembranosus

transversus abdominis*

rectus femoris

gastrocnemius

Annotation Key
* indicates deep muscles

teres minor

teres major

serratus anterior

obliquus externus

pectoralis major

deltoideus posterior

trapezius

deltoideus anterior

obliquus internus*

rectus abdominis

biceps brachii

triceps brachii

vastus medialis

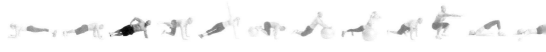

Side Plank

Side Plank stabilizes your spine, but it is also great for strengthening your abdominals, lower back, and shoulders.

1 Lie on your left side with your legs straight and parallel to each other. Keep your feet flexed.

2 Bend your left arm to a 90-degree angle with the knuckles of your hand facing forward. Place your right hand on your waist or extend your arm along your side.

3 Pressing your forearm down into the floor, raise your hips until your body is in a straight line. Hold for 30 seconds, working up to 1 minute. Repeat on the other side.

Correct form
· Push evenly from both your forearm and hips.

Avoid
· Placing too much strain on your shoulders; they should neither sink into their sockets nor lift toward your ears.

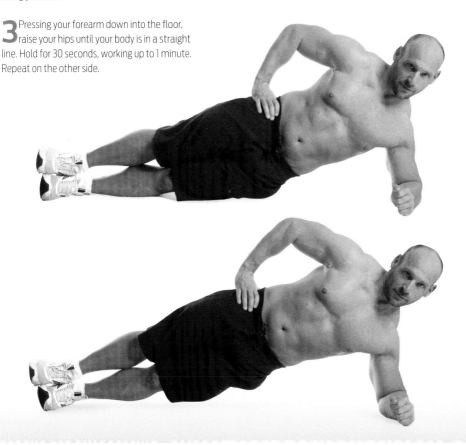

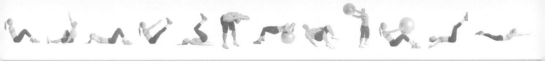

Diary of practice

	Date	Time held	Comment
Week 1			
Week 2			
Week 3			
Week 4			

Annotation Key
* indicates deep muscles

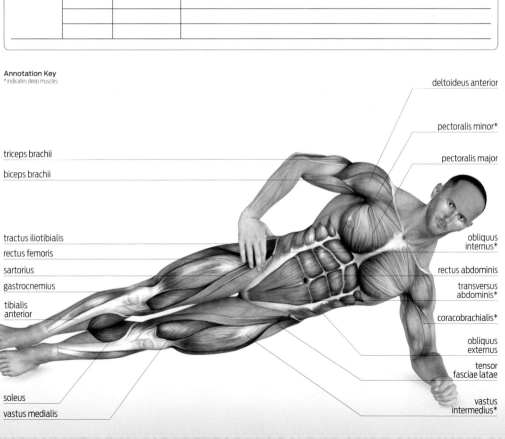

deltoideus anterior

pectoralis minor*

pectoralis major

triceps brachii

biceps brachii

obliquus internus*

rectus abdominis

tractus iliotibialis

rectus femoris

sartorius

transversus abdominis*

gastrocnemius

tibialis anterior

coracobrachialis*

obliquus externus

tensor fasciae latae

soleus

vastus medialis

vastus intermedius*

 DVD section 2: Chapter 6

Fire Hydrant In-Out

Fire Hydrant In-Out is a hard-working core-stabilizing exercise, as well as a great core-strengthener. It targets your inner thighs, hamstrings, and glutes, with assistance from your abdominal muscles.

1 Begin on your hands and knees, with your palms on the floor and spaced shoulder-width apart. Your spine should be in a neutral position.

2 Keeping your right leg bent at a 90-degree angle, raise it laterally, or to the side.

3 Straighten your right leg until it is fully extended behind you so that it is in line with your torso.

4 Bend your right knee and bring your leg back into its 90-degree position, and then lower it to meet your left leg. Work up to 15 repetitions. Repeat on the other side.

Correct form
· Press your hands into the floor to keep your shoulders from sinking.
· Squeeze your gluteal muscles with your leg fully extended.

Avoid
· Lifting your hip as you lift your bent leg to the side.
· Rushing through the exercise; make sure that you feel each portion of the repetition.

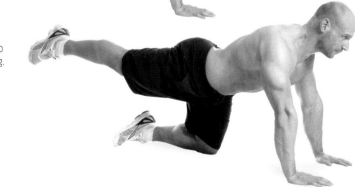

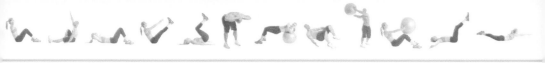

Diary of practice

	Date	Repetitions	Comment
Week 1			
Week 2			
Week 3			
Week 4			

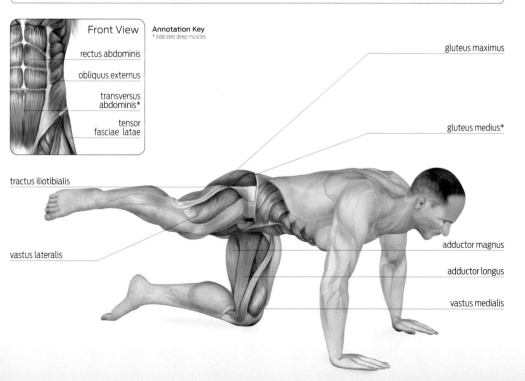

Front View

rectus abdominis
obliquus externus
transversus abdominis*
tensor fasciae latae

Annotation Key
* indicates deep muscles

gluteus maximus

gluteus medius*

tractus iliotibialis

vastus lateralis

adductor magnus

adductor longus

vastus medialis

 DVD section 2: Chapter 7

T-Stabilization

T-Stabilization, another advanced variation on the traditional Plank, is a proven exercise for targeting your abs, hips, lower back, and obliques.

1 Assume the finished push-up position with your arms extended to full lockout, your fingers facing forward, your legs outstretched, and your body weight supported on your toes.

2 Turn your hips to one side, collapsing one foot on top of the other and raising your top arm across your body until you are pointing toward the ceiling.

3 Hold for 30 seconds, lower, and then repeat on the other side. Work your way up to holding for 1 minute on each side.

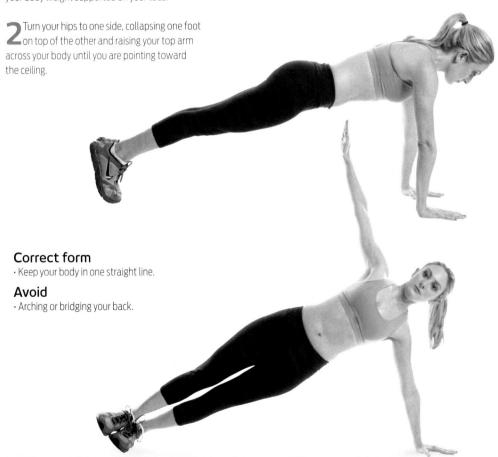

Correct form
· Keep your body in one straight line.

Avoid
· Arching or bridging your back.

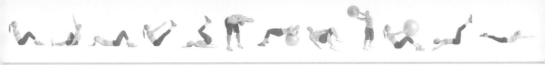

Diary of practice

	Date	Time held	Comment
Week 1			
Week 2			
Week 3			
Week 4			

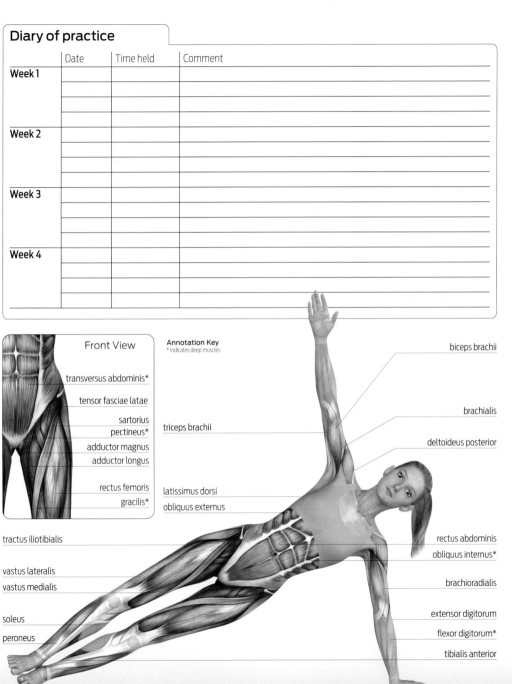

Front View

Annotation Key
* indicates deep muscles

transversus abdominis*
tensor fasciae latae
sartorius
pectineus*
adductor magnus
adductor longus
rectus femoris
gracilis*

triceps brachii

latissimus dorsi
obliquus externus

tractus iliotibialis

vastus lateralis
vastus medialis

soleus

peroneus

biceps brachii

brachialis

deltoideus posterior

rectus abdominis
obliquus internus*

brachioradialis

extensor digitorum
flexor digitorum*

tibialis anterior

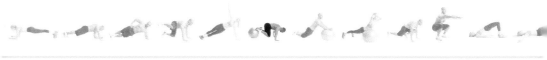

 DVD section 2: Chapter 8

Fitness Ball Atomic Push-Up

Performing the Fitness Ball Atomic Push-Up causes many major muscle groups to fire at once. When executed properly, this exercise tones your upper body, engages your core, and works your hip flexors.

1 Begin on your hands and knees with your fingers facing forward and a fitness ball placed behind you. Rest your shins on the ball, and straighten your legs so that your body forms a straight line.

2 While keeping your back flat, bend your knees to draw the fitness ball into your core.

3 Straighten your legs, moving the ball farther behind you, and then perform a push-up. Start with 5 repetitions, working your way up to 2 sets of 12 to 15.

Correct form
· Keep your hips level with your torso.

Avoid
· Piking or bridging your body.

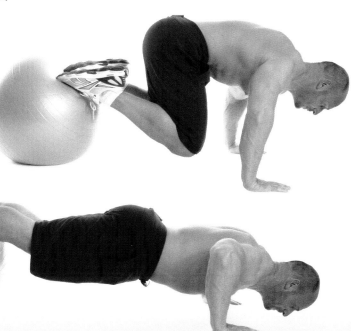

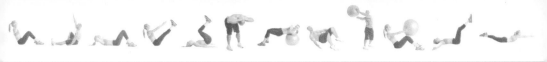

Diary of practice

	Date	Repetitions	Comment
Week 1			
Week 2			
Week 3			
Week 4			

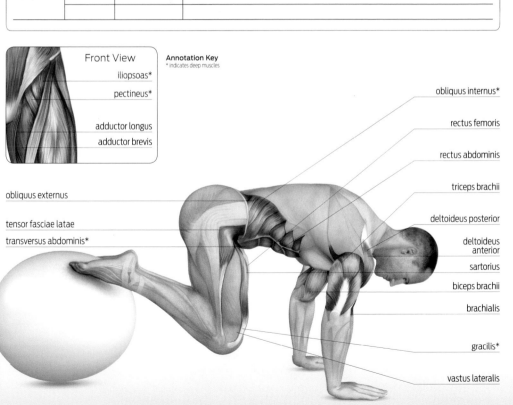

Front View

iliopsoas*
pectineus*
adductor longus
adductor brevis

Annotation Key
* indicates deep muscles

obliquus internus*
rectus femoris
rectus abdominis
triceps brachii
deltoideus posterior
deltoideus anterior
sartorius
biceps brachii
brachialis
gracilis*
vastus lateralis

obliquus externus
tensor fasciae latae
transversus abdominis*

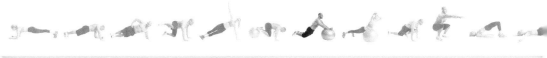

 DVD section 2: Chapter 9

Fitness Ball Rollout

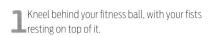

Fitness Ball Rollout is a fun and challenging exercise for effectively stabilizing your core. Aim for controlled, steady movement throughout.

1 Kneel behind your fitness ball, with your fists resting on top of it.

2 Extend the ball forward, leading with your arms and following with your body until you are completely stretched out while maintaining a flat back and staying anchored on your knees.

3 Using your abdominals and lower back, roll back in until you reach an upright position. Work up to 3 sets of 15 repetitions.

Correct form
· Keep your body elongated throughout the movement.

Avoid
· Bridging your back and allowing your hips to sag.

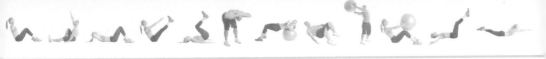

Diary of practice

	Date	Repetitions	Comment
Week 1			
Week 2			
Week 3			
Week 4			

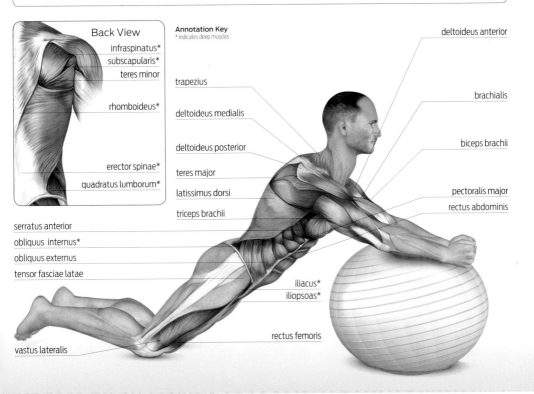

Back View

infraspinatus*
subscapularis*
teres minor

rhomboideus*

erector spinae*
quadratus lumborum*

Annotation Key
* indicates deep muscles

trapezius

deltoideus medialis

deltoideus posterior

teres major

latissimus dorsi

triceps brachii

serratus anterior
obliquus internus*
obliquus externus
tensor fasciae latae

iliacus*
iliopsoas*

rectus femoris

vastus lateralis

deltoideus anterior

brachialis

biceps brachii

pectoralis major
rectus abdominis

Fitness Ball Hyperextension

Fitness Ball Hyperextension, executed on the large fitness ball, is a safe and effective alternative to traditional hyperextension machines. Performing this exercise is a great way to work your lower-back muscles.

1 Begin in a facedown position on top of the fitness ball, with your abdominals covering most of the ball, your legs spread with toes on the floor, and your arms behind your head. Push your toes into the floor for stability.

2 Raise your torso so that it forms a line with the lower half of your body.

3 Squeeze your gluteal muscles as you lower your upper body, and then raise it back to the starting position. Continue lowering and raising, working up to 3 sets of 15 to 20 repetitions.

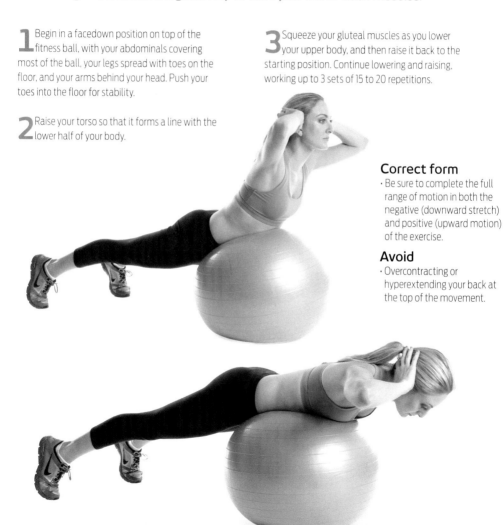

Correct form
· Be sure to complete the full range of motion in both the negative (downward stretch) and positive (upward motion) of the exercise.

Avoid
· Overcontracting or hyperextending your back at the top of the movement.

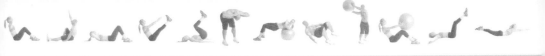

Diary of practice

	Date	Repetitions	Comment
Week 1			
Week 2			
Week 3			
Week 4			

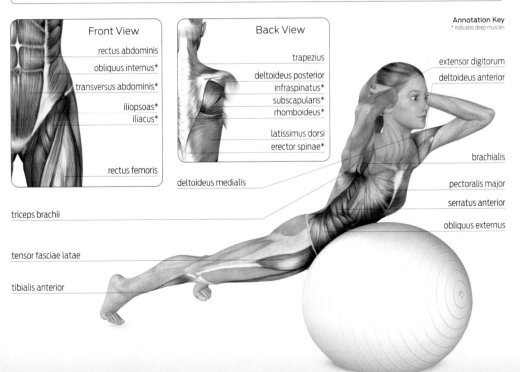

Front View

rectus abdominis
obliquus internus*
transversus abdominis*
iliopsoas*
iliacus*
rectus femoris

triceps brachii

tensor fasciae latae

tibialis anterior

Back View

trapezius
deltoideus posterior
infraspinatus*
subscapularis*
rhomboideus*
latissimus dorsi
erector spinae*
deltoideus medialis

Annotation Key
* indicates deep muscles

extensor digitorum
deltoideus anterior

brachialis

pectoralis major
serratus anterior
obliquus externus

 DVD section 2: Chapter 11

Mountain Climber

Mountain Climber is a core-stabilizing, timed distance exercise. This high-intensity move gets your heart rate going, improving your cardiovascular fitness, while it challenges your legs and core. This all-around exercise also helps to develop muscular endurance in your arms.

1 Begin in a completed push-up position with your body forming a straight line.

2 Bend one knee and bring it as close to your chest as possible.

3 Return to the starting position and repeat with your other leg. Continue to alternate for 30 seconds, working up to 2 minutes.

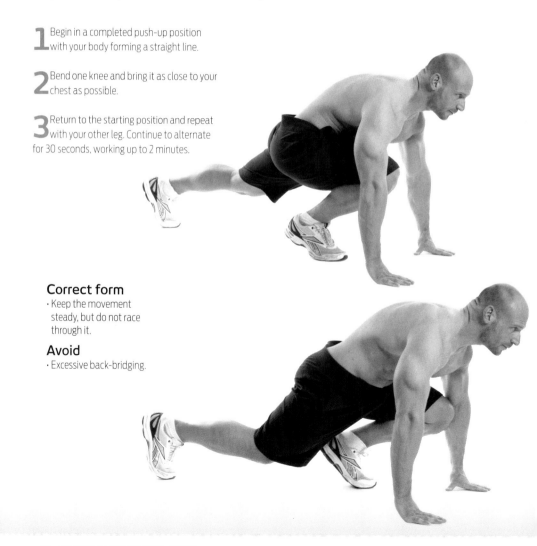

Correct form
· Keep the movement steady, but do not race through it.

Avoid
· Excessive back-bridging.

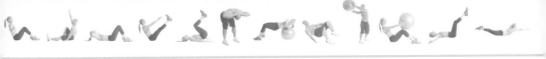

Diary of practice

	Date	Repetitions	Comment
Week 1			
Week 2			
Week 3			
Week 4			

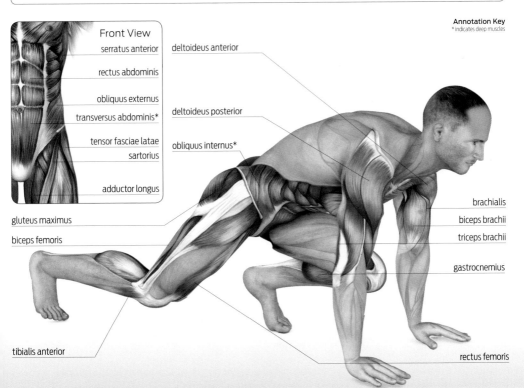

Annotation Key
* indicates deep muscles

Front View

serratus anterior

rectus abdominis

obliquus externus

transversus abdominis*

tensor fasciae latae

sartorius

adductor longus

gluteus maximus

biceps femoris

tibialis anterior

deltoideus anterior

deltoideus posterior

obliquus internus*

brachialis

biceps brachii

triceps brachii

gastrocnemius

rectus femoris

Body-Weight Squat

Body-Weight Squat is a full-body exercise. Completing it correctly means using your core properly. It may look like an easy move, but there is more to it: as well as engaging your leg muscles, it engages nearly every muscle in your lower body. Perfecting this exercise is a great way to combat the weakness that often develops from a sedentary lifestyle.

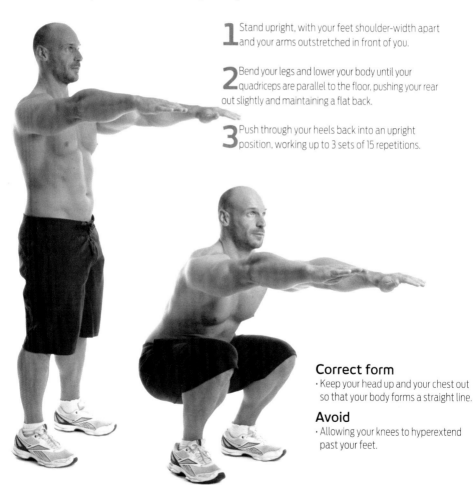

1 Stand upright, with your feet shoulder-width apart and your arms outstretched in front of you.

2 Bend your legs and lower your body until your quadriceps are parallel to the floor, pushing your rear out slightly and maintaining a flat back.

3 Push through your heels back into an upright position, working up to 3 sets of 15 repetitions.

Correct form
· Keep your head up and your chest out so that your body forms a straight line.

Avoid
· Allowing your knees to hyperextend past your feet.

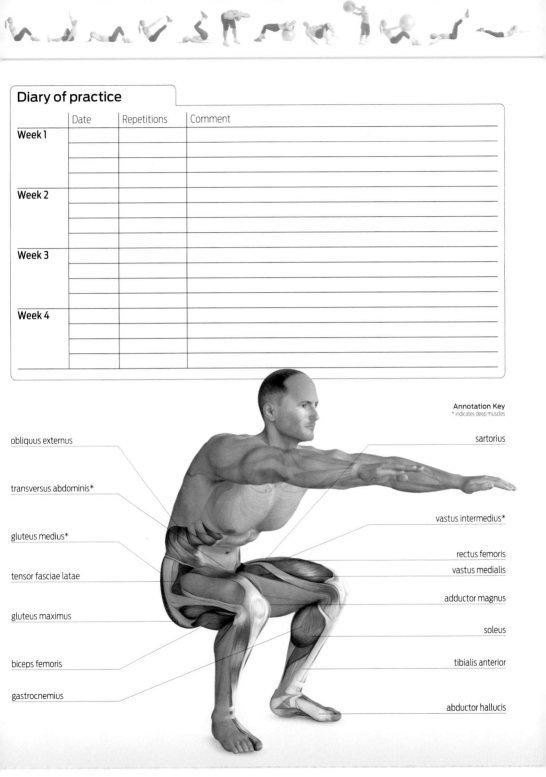

Diary of practice

	Date	Repetitions	Comment
Week 1			
Week 2			
Week 3			
Week 4			

Annotation Key
* indicates deep muscles

obliquus externus

transversus abdominis*

gluteus medius*

tensor fasciae latae

gluteus maximus

biceps femoris

gastrocnemius

sartorius

vastus intermedius*

rectus femoris

vastus medialis

adductor magnus

soleus

tibialis anterior

abductor hallucis

 DVD section 2: Chapter 13

Hip Raise

Adding movement to the traditional Shoulder Bridge, Hip Raise really challenges your core strength. It is not only an abdominal and lower-back exercise, but it also targets your gluteal and hamstring muscles.

1 Lie on your back with your legs bent, your feet flat on the floor, and your arms along your sides.

2 Push through your heels while raising your pelvis until your torso is aligned with your thighs. Lower and then repeat, working up to 3 sets of 15.

Correct form
· Push through your heels, not your toes.

Avoid
· Overextending your abdominals past your thighs in the raised position.

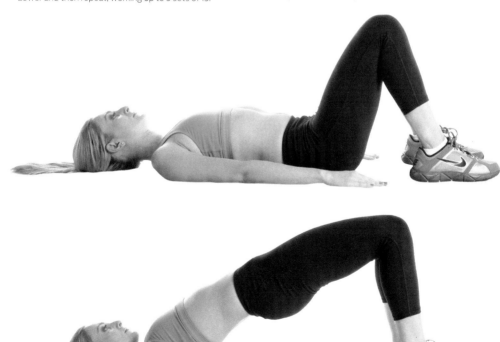

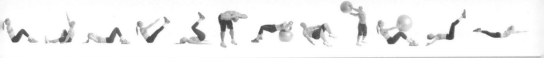

Diary of practice

	Date	Repetitions	Comment
Week 1			
Week 2			
Week 3			
Week 4			

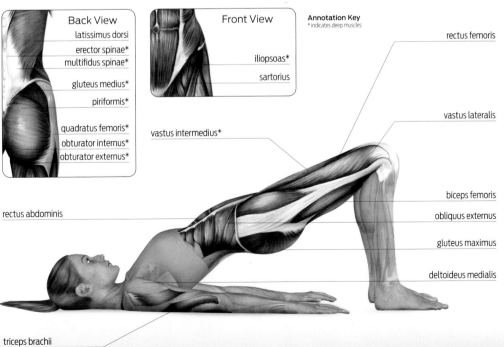

Back View
- latissimus dorsi
- erector spinae*
- multifidus spinae*
- gluteus medius*
- piriformis*
- quadratus femoris*
- obturator internus*
- obturator externus*

Front View
- iliopsoas*
- sartorius

Annotation Key
* indicates deep muscles

- rectus femoris
- vastus lateralis
- biceps femoris
- obliquus externus
- gluteus maximus
- deltoideus medialis

- vastus intermedius*
- rectus abdominis
- triceps brachii

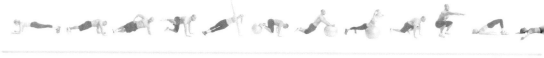

Hip Crossover

Hip Crossover effectively targets your lower-back and oblique muscles. As with many core exercises, when executing Hip Crossover, look for controlled movements. You want your muscles to move you—not momentum.

1 Lie on your back with your arms lengthened away from your body and your legs bent at a 90-degree angle and lifted off the floor.

2 Brace your abs and lower your knees to the side, dropping them as close to the floor as possible without lifting your shoulders off the mat.

3 Return to the starting position, hold for a moment, and then repeat on the other side. Work up to 15 repetitions per side.

Correct form
· Keep your core centered.

Avoid
· Excessively swinging your legs; you want to move carefully and with control.

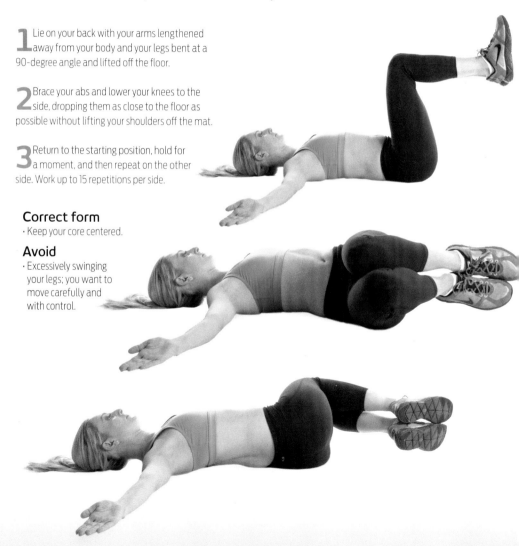

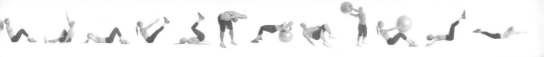

Diary of practice

	Date	Repetitions	Comment
Week 1			
Week 2			
Week 3			
Week 4			

Annotation Key
* indicates deep muscles

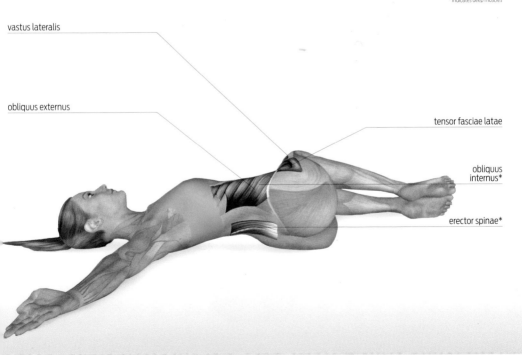

vastus lateralis

obliquus externus

tensor fasciae latae

obliquus internus*

erector spinae*

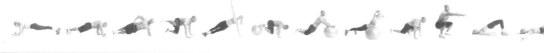

 DVD section 2: Chapter 15

Sit-Up

The Sit-Up is a basic exercise for both strengthening and defining the abdominal muscles. This workout staple also works the hip flexor muscles. Form is crucial; improperly performed Sit-Ups can strain your spine and the muscles in your head and neck.

1 Lie on your back with your legs bent and your feet firmly planted on the floor. Your hands should be behind your head, your elbows flared outward.

2 Raise your shoulders and torso off the floor toward your legs. Lower and repeat, working up to 3 sets of 20.

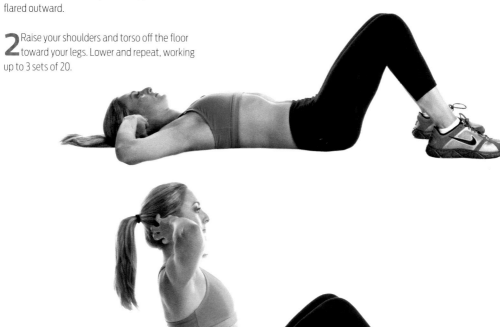

Correct form
· Lead with your abdominals, not with your neck.

Avoid
· Using excessive momentum.
· Overusing your lower back.

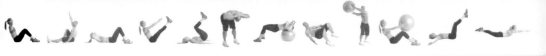

Diary of practice

	Date	Repetitions	Comment
Week 1			
Week 2			
Week 3			
Week 4			

Annotation Key
* indicates deep muscles

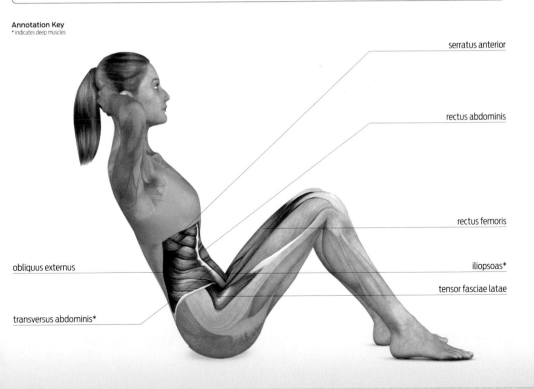

serratus anterior

rectus abdominis

rectus femoris

obliquus externus

iliopsoas*

tensor fasciae latae

transversus abdominis*

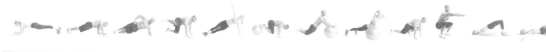

 DVD section 2: Chapter 16

One-Armed Sit-Up

One-Armed Sit-Up is a challenging twist on the traditional Sit-Up, engaging the obliques and the latissimus dorsi, as well as the rectus abdominis.

1 Lie on your back with your left leg bent and your right leg lengthened along the floor. Extend your left arm behind your head, and rest your right arm along your side.

2 Pushing through your left heel, raise your shoulders and torso off the floor until you are sitting nearly upright and your left arm is directly over your head. Lower and repeat on the other side, working up to 2 sets of 15 repetitions.

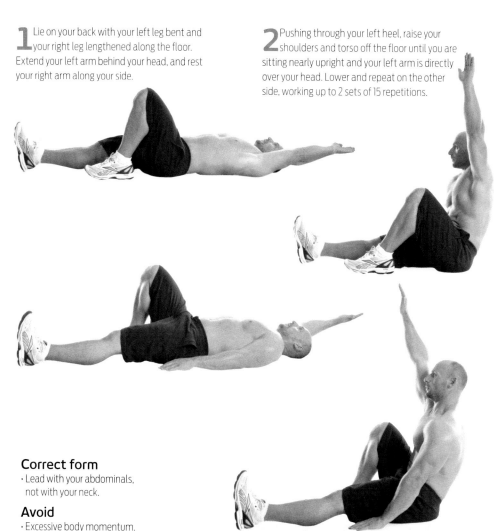

Correct form
· Lead with your abdominals, not with your neck.

Avoid
· Excessive body momentum.
· Overusing your lower back.

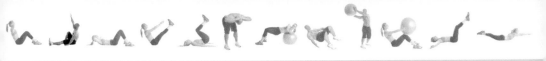

Diary of practice

	Date	Repetitions	Comment
Week 1			
Week 2			
Week 3			
Week 4			

Annotation Key
* indicates deep muscles

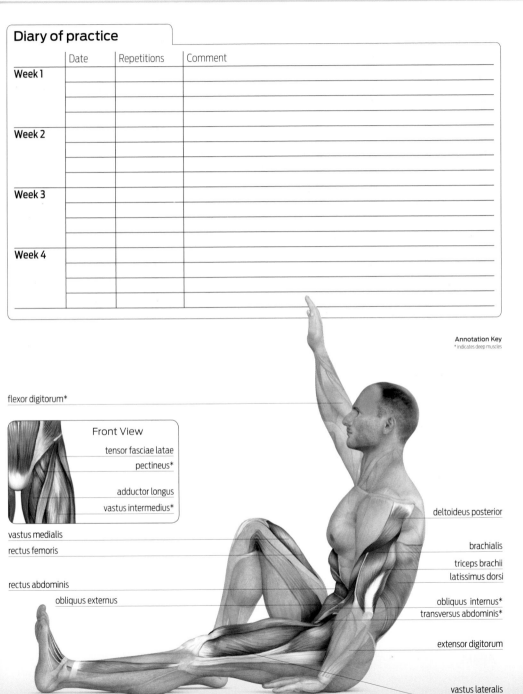

flexor digitorum*

Front View

tensor fasciae latae
pectineus*

adductor longus
vastus intermedius*

vastus medialis
rectus femoris

rectus abdominis
obliquus externus

deltoideus posterior

brachialis
triceps brachii
latissimus dorsi

obliquus internus*
transversus abdominis*

extensor digitorum

vastus lateralis

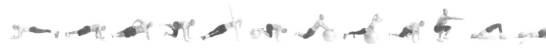

Crunch

Like the Sit-Up, the Crunch is highly effective for isolating the rectus abdominis. Unlike the Sit-Up, however, your lower back never leaves the floor during the movement, which places less strain on the lumbar region of your spine.

1 Lie on your back with your legs bent, elbows flared, and palms next to your ears.

2 Raise your head and shoulders off the floor while contracting your abdominals. Lower and repeat, working up to 3 sets of 25 repetitions.

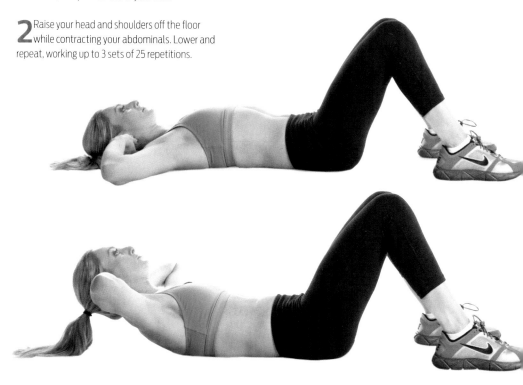

Correct form
· Lead with your abdominals, as if a string were hoisting you up by your belly button.

Avoid
· Overusing your neck.

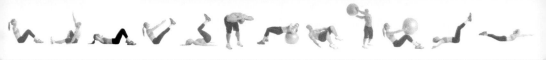

Diary of practice

	Date	Repetitions	Comment
Week 1			
Week 2			
Week 3			
Week 4			

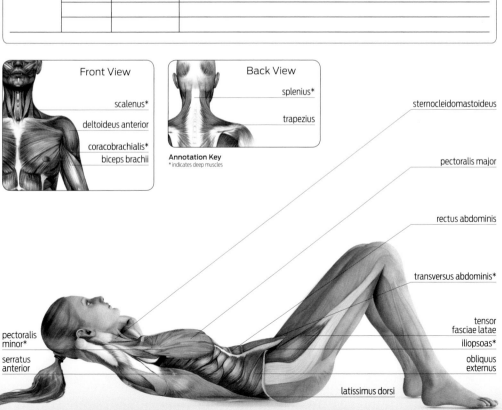

Front View

scalenus*
deltoideus anterior
coracobrachialis*
biceps brachii

Back View

splenius*
trapezius

Annotation Key
* indicates deep muscles

sternocleidomastoideus

pectoralis major

rectus abdominis

transversus abdominis*

tensor
fasciae latae
iliopsoas*

obliquus
externus

pectoralis
minor*

serratus
anterior

latissimus dorsi

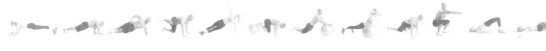

DVD section 2: Chapter 18

V-Up

The challenging V-Up targets both your upper and lower rectus abdominis as it moves through its entire range of motion. Performing V-Ups is also an efficient way to strengthen your lower-back muscles and tighten your quads.

1 Lie on your back with your arms and legs elongated on the floor.

2 Simultaneously raise your arms and legs so that your arms are nearly touching your feet, while maintaining a flat back. Lower and repeat, working up to 3 sets of 20 repetitions.

Correct form
· Keep your arms and legs straight.

Avoid
· Using a jerking motion as your raise or lower your arms and legs.

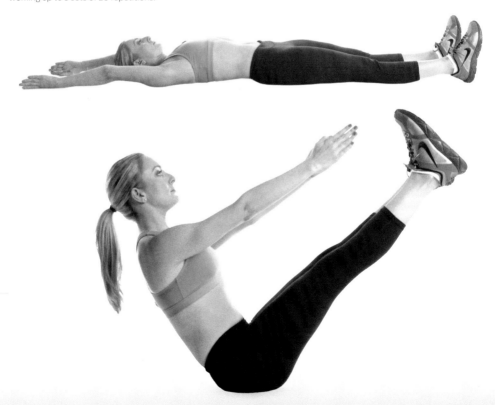

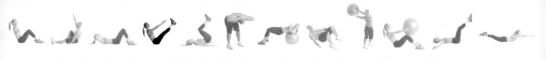

Diary of practice

	Date	Repetitions	Comment
Week 1			
Week 2			
Week 3			
Week 4			

Annotation Key
* indicates deep muscles

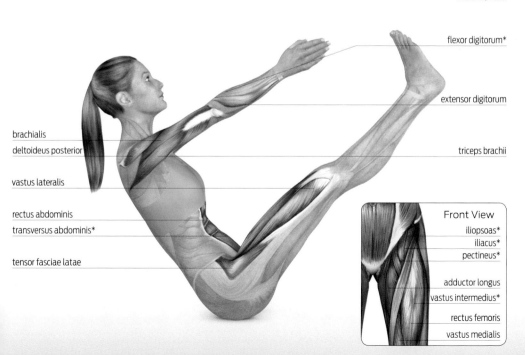

flexor digitorum*

extensor digitorum

triceps brachii

brachialis

deltoideus posterior

vastus lateralis

rectus abdominis

transversus abdominis*

tensor fasciae latae

Front View
iliopsoas*
iliacus*
pectineus*

adductor longus
vastus intermedius*
rectus femoris
vastus medialis

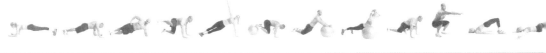

 DVD section 2: Chapter 19

Reverse Crunch

The Reverse Crunch is highly effective for isolating the lowest portion of the rectus abdominis, where most abdominal fat tends to be stored. Less is more with this exercise: your movements should be small but focused.

1 Lie on your back with your arms at your sides and your legs bent at a 90-degree angle with your feet off the floor.

2 Lift your buttocks a few inches off the mat as you bring your knees toward your chest. Lower in a controlled manner. Repeat, working up to 3 sets of 20 repetitions.

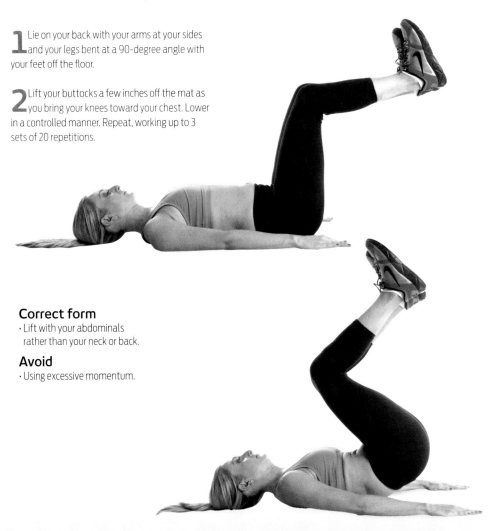

Correct form
· Lift with your abdominals rather than your neck or back.

Avoid
· Using excessive momentum.

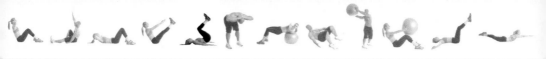

Diary of practice

	Date	Repetitions	Comment
Week 1			
Week 2			
Week 3			
Week 4			

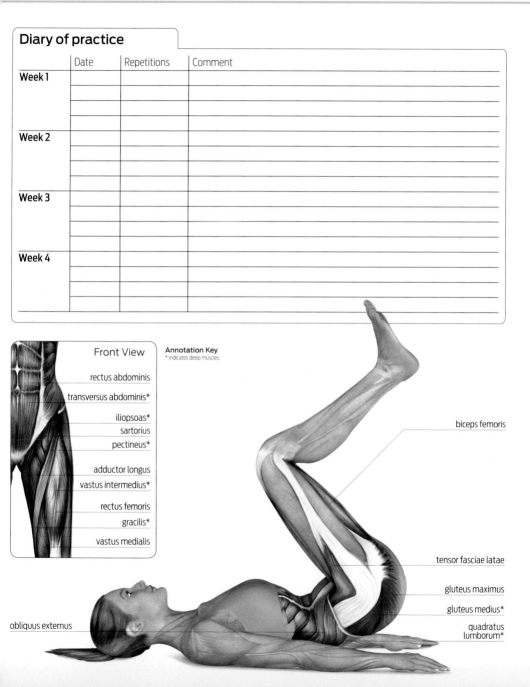

Front View

Annotation Key
* indicates deep muscles

rectus abdominis

transversus abdominis*

iliopsoas*

sartorius

pectineus*

adductor longus

vastus intermedius*

rectus femoris

gracilis*

vastus medialis

biceps femoris

tensor fasciae latae

gluteus maximus

gluteus medius*

quadratus lumborum*

obliquus externus

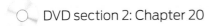
Good Mornings

Good Mornings are effective moves for strengthening your lower back. Weight lifters commonly use a barbell to perform Good Mornings, but here your own body weight provides the resistance for the exercise.

1 Stand upright with your hands clasped behind your head, elbows flared out, and feet shoulder-width apart.

2 Bend your knees slightly and stick your rear out while hinging forward from the waist until your back is nearly parallel to the floor. Return to an upright position and repeat, working up to 3 sets of 15 repetitions.

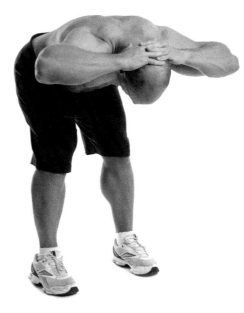

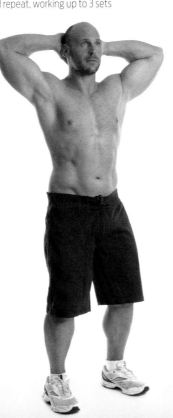

Correct form
· Perform the exercise slowly and with control.

Avoid
· Rounding your back.

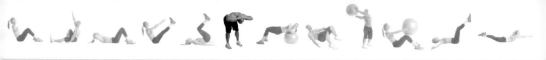

Diary of practice

	Date	Repetitions	Comment
Week 1			
Week 2			
Week 3			
Week 4			

erector spinae*

latissimus dorsi

Annotation Key
* indicates deep muscles

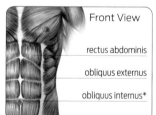

Front View

rectus abdominis

obliquus externus

obliquus internus*

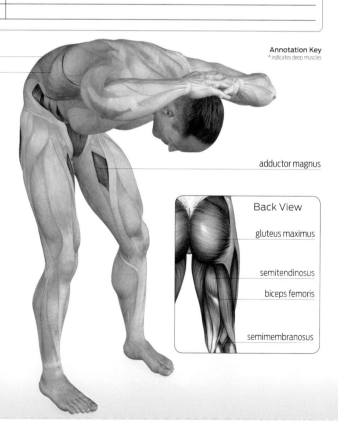

adductor magnus

Back View

gluteus maximus

semitendinosus

biceps femoris

semimembranosus

 DVD section 2: Chapter 21

Fitness Ball Russian Twist

Fitness Ball Russian Twist offers a fun, unique way to strengthen your core—and whittle your waistline. It targets all of your abdominals, but because it incorporates rotation, it places an emphasis on the obliques.

1 Sit on your fitness ball, with feet planted shoulder-width apart. Roll forward until your neck is supported on the ball. Extend your arms to full lockout directly above your chest.

2 Turn one hip out to the side while also turning your torso and your arms. Return to the center and repeat on the other side, working up to 3 sets of 15 repetitions per side.

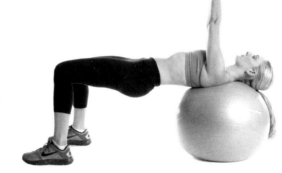

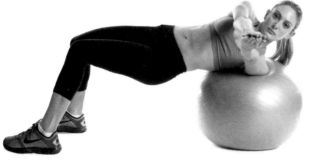

Correct form
· Move slowly and with control.

Avoid
· Allowing your upper back to hang off the fitness ball, unsupported.

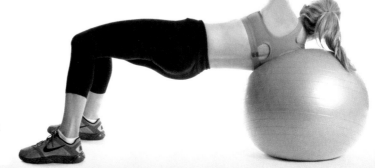

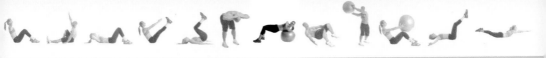

Diary of practice

	Date	Repetitions	Comment
Week 1			
Week 2			
Week 3			
Week 4			

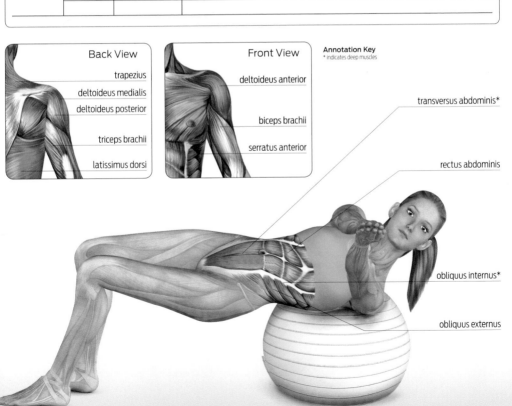

Back View

trapezius

deltoideus medialis

deltoideus posterior

triceps brachii

latissimus dorsi

Front View

deltoideus anterior

biceps brachii

serratus anterior

Annotation Key
* indicates deep muscles

transversus abdominis*

rectus abdominis

obliquus internus*

obliquus externus

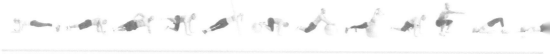

 DVD section 2: Chapter 22

Penguin Crunch

Penguin Crunch, also called the Penguin Heel Reach, targets your oblique muscles. Because it incorporates lateral movement of the abdominals, it is a great exercise to prepare you for any sport that requires rotational movement, such as swimming or diving.

1 Begin on your back, with your head elevated and your arms at your sides and raised off the floor.

2 Reach forward in a stabbing motion with one hand, and then pull back. Lower and repeat with the other hand, working up to 3 sets of 15 repetitions on each side.

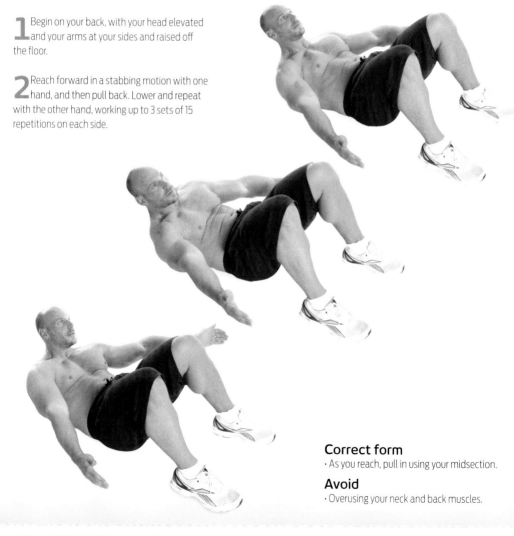

Correct form
· As you reach, pull in using your midsection.

Avoid
· Overusing your neck and back muscles.

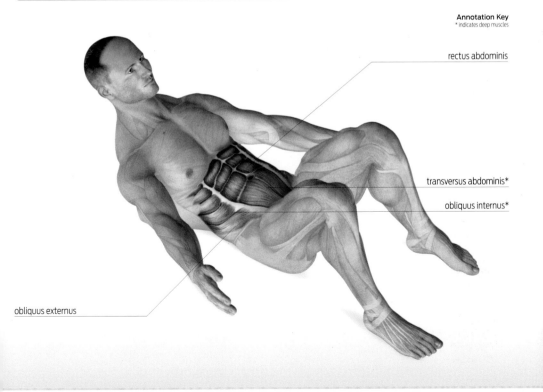

Diary of practice

	Date	Repetitions	Comment
Week 1			
Week 2			
Week 3			
Week 4			

Annotation Key
* indicates deep muscles

rectus abdominis

transversus abdominis*

obliquus internus*

obliquus externus

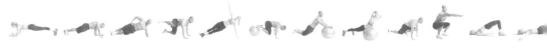

 DVD section 2: Chapter 23

Wood Chop with Fitness Ball

Wood Chop with Fitness Ball is another take on a gym classic. Perform this version of the Wood Chop to strengthen your abdominals, especially the oblique muscles. This exercise also works your arm and shoulder muscles.

1 Stand up while holding your large fitness ball. Twist your core to one side, bringing the ball with you.

2 Lower the ball, and then follow through by twisting to the other side and raising it as you turn, as if swinging a baseball bat, while feeling your core contract. Lower the ball. Repeat through the same range of motion on the other side, working up to 3 sets of 20 per side.

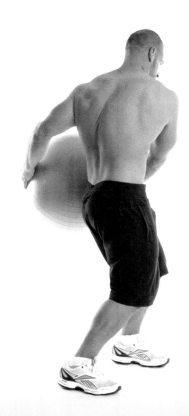

Correct form
· Perform the swinging portion of the exercise aggressively, and the wind-up portion more slowly.
· Keep your core contracted and tight throughout.

Avoid
· Straining your back by twisting too vigorously from side to side.

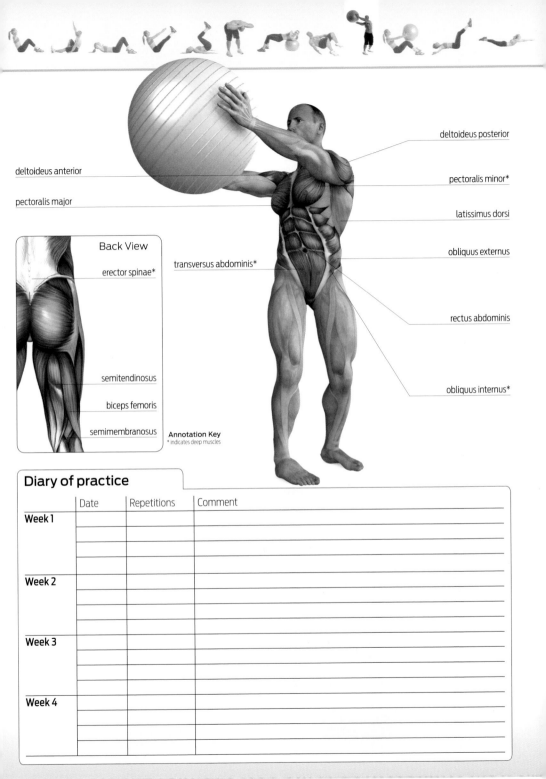

deltoideus posterior

deltoideus anterior

pectoralis minor*

pectoralis major

latissimus dorsi

obliquus externus

Back View

transversus abdominis*

erector spinae*

rectus abdominis

semitendinosus

biceps femoris

obliquus internus*

semimembranosus

Annotation Key
* indicates deep muscles

Diary of practice

	Date	Repetitions	Comment
Week 1			
Week 2			
Week 3			
Week 4			

Fitness Ball Seated Russian Twist

Fitness Ball Seated Russian Twist is effective for strengthening the major muscles of your core, including your obliques, lower-back extensors, abdominals, and deep core stabilizers.

1 Begin seated with your legs apart while holding a fitness ball at arms' length. Lean back slightly to activate your core.

2 While keeping a flat back, begin rotating from side to side. Work up to performing 3 sets of 20 rotations.

Correct form
· Twist with control, and not too speedily.

Avoid
· Rounding your back.

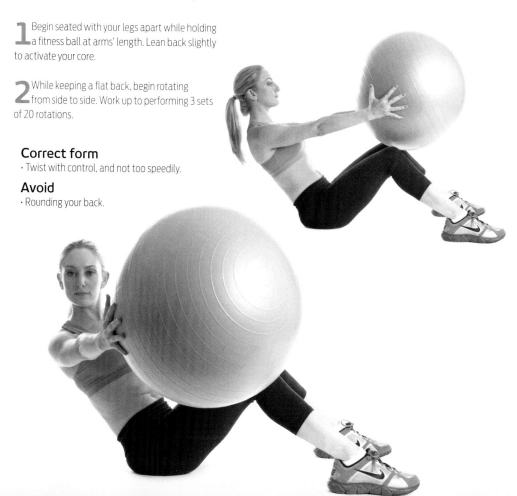

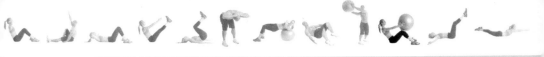

Diary of practice

	Date	Repetitions	Comment
Week 1			
Week 2			
Week 3			
Week 4			

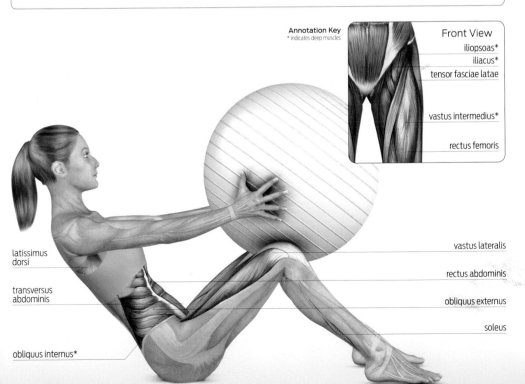

Annotation Key
* indicates deep muscles

Front View

iliopsoas*
iliacus*
tensor fasciae latae
vastus intermedius*
rectus femoris

latissimus dorsi

transversus abdominis

obliquus internus*

vastus lateralis

rectus abdominis

obliquus externus

soleus

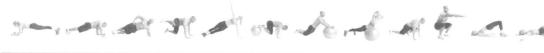

 DVD section 2: Chapter 25

Leg Raises

Leg Raises target the transversus abdominis: that tough-to-reach lower abdominal area. This core-strengthening exercise is easy do to, even for most beginners. Perform it regularly to see a reduction in abdominal fat.

1 Lie on your back with your arms out at your sides. Bend your legs slightly and elevate them off the floor.

2 Lower your legs to just above floor level, lift them back up, and repeat. Work up to performing 2 sets of 20 repetitions.

Correct form
· Keep your upper body braced.

Avoid
· Using momentum or your lower back to drive the movement.

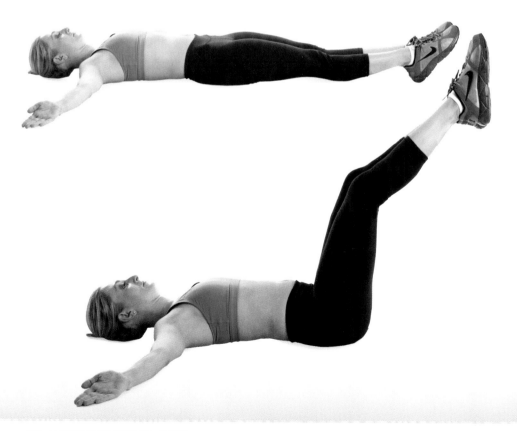

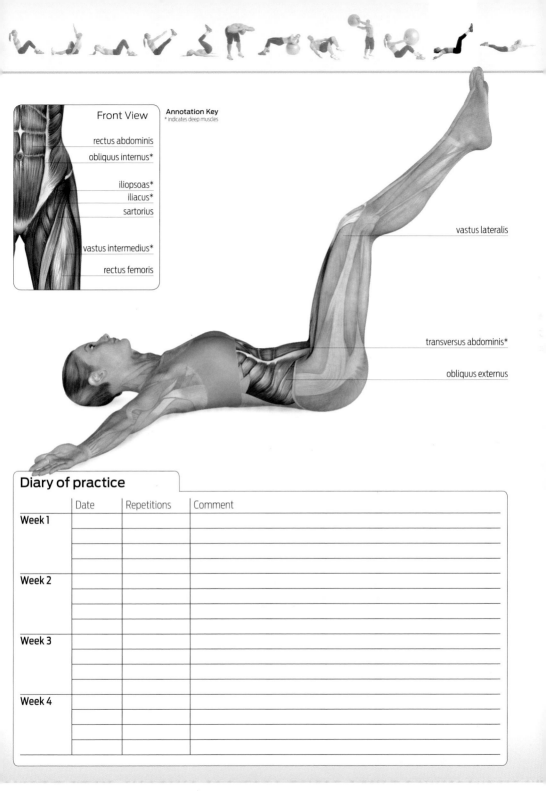

rectus abdominis

obliquus internus*

iliopsoas*
iliacus*
sartorius

vastus intermedius*

rectus femoris

vastus lateralis

transversus abdominis*

obliquus externus

Diary of practice

	Date	Repetitions	Comment
Week 1			
Week 2			
Week 3			
Week 4			

○ DVD section 2: Chapter 26

Superman

Superman is great for targeting your entire core as well as your hip flexors and legs extended on the floor. It is also an effective exercise for your back, strengthening both the full extent of the erector spinae, as well as the multifidus spinae. Beware though—this move is harder than it looks.

1 Lie facedown on your stomach with your arms and legs extended on the floor.

2 Raise your arms and your legs simultaneously, squeezing your glutes at the top, and then lower. Work up to 3 sets of 15.

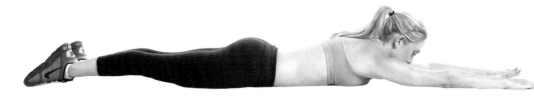

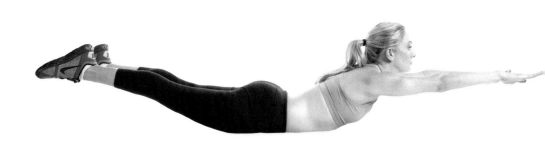

Correct form
· Raise your arms and legs as high as possible.

Avoid
· Overstressing your neck.

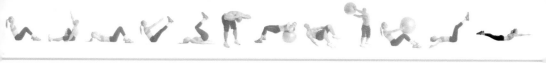

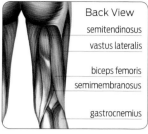

Back View

semitendinosus

vastus lateralis

biceps femoris
semimembranosus

gastrocnemius

Annotation Key
* indicates deep muscles

Back View

semispinalis*
splenius*
trapezius

infraspinatus*
teres minor
teres major
rhomboideus*

latissimus dorsi

erector spinae*
quadratus lumborum*

Front View

sternocleidomastoideus

scalenus*
deltoideus medialis

deltoideus anterior

biceps brachii

flexor digitorum*

extensor
carpi radialis

deltoideus posterior

gluteus maximus

triceps brachii

peroneus

tibialis anterior

rectus femoris
vastus intermedius*

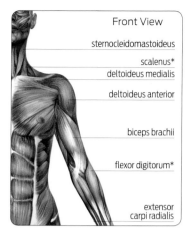

Diary of practice

	Date	Repetitions	Comment
Week 1			
Week 2			
Week 3			
Week 4			

Full-Body Anatomy

Front View

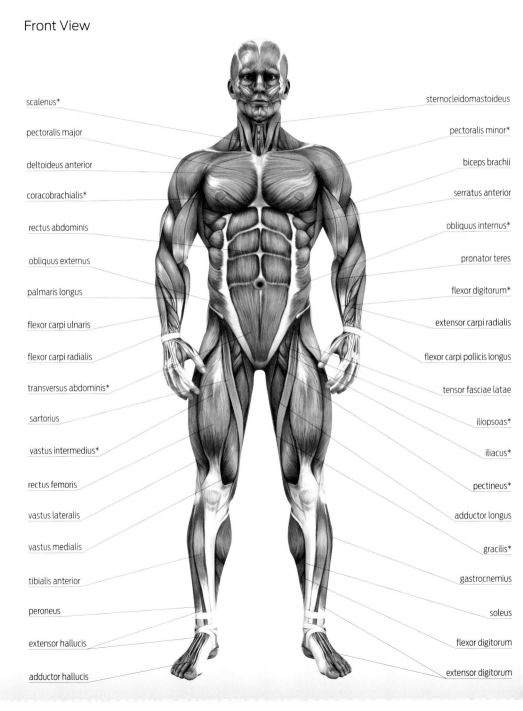

scalenus*

pectoralis major

deltoideus anterior

coracobrachialis*

rectus abdominis

obliquus externus

palmaris longus

flexor carpi ulnaris

flexor carpi radialis

transversus abdominis*

sartorius

vastus intermedius*

rectus femoris

vastus lateralis

vastus medialis

tibialis anterior

peroneus

extensor hallucis

adductor hallucis

sternocleidomastoideus

pectoralis minor*

biceps brachii

serratus anterior

obliquus internus*

pronator teres

flexor digitorum*

extensor carpi radialis

flexor carpi pollicis longus

tensor fasciae latae

iliopsoas*

iliacus*

pectineus*

adductor longus

gracilis*

gastrocnemius

soleus

flexor digitorum

extensor digitorum

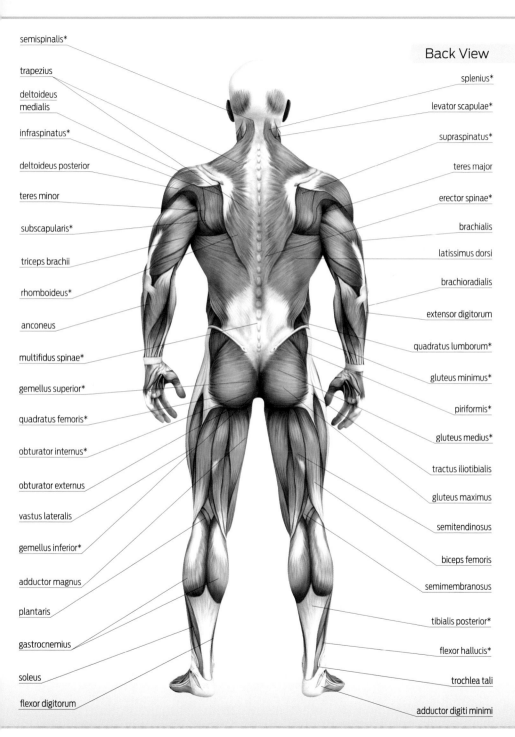

semispinalis*

trapezius

deltoideus
medialis

infraspinatus*

deltoideus posterior

teres minor

subscapularis*

triceps brachii

rhomboideus*

anconeus

multifidus spinae*

gemellus superior*

quadratus femoris*

obturator internus*

obturator externus

vastus lateralis

gemellus inferior*

adductor magnus

plantaris

gastrocnemius

soleus

flexor digitorum

splenius*

levator scapulae*

supraspinatus*

teres major

erector spinae*

brachialis

latissimus dorsi

brachioradialis

extensor digitorum

quadratus lumborum*

gluteus minimus*

piriformis*

gluteus medius*

tractus iliotibialis

gluteus maximus

semitendinosus

biceps femoris

semimembranosus

tibialis posterior*

flexor hallucis*

trochlea tali

adductor digiti minimi

Targeted Workouts

Beginner's Workout
Suitable for all levels, this workout is great for beginners new to core training.

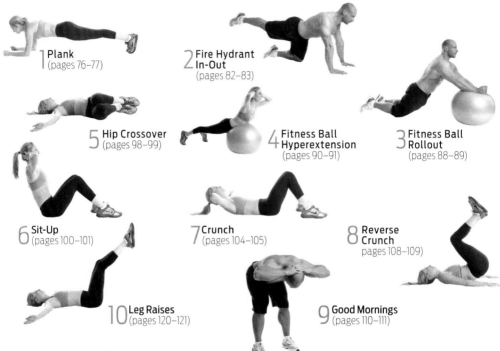

1 **Plank**
(pages 76–77)

2 **Fire Hydrant In-Out**
(pages 82–83)

5 **Hip Crossover**
(pages 98–99)

4 **Fitness Ball Hyperextension**
(pages 90–91)

3 **Fitness Ball Rollout**
(pages 88–89)

6 **Sit-Up**
(pages 100–101)

7 **Crunch**
(pages 104–105)

8 **Reverse Crunch**
pages 108–109)

10 **Leg Raises**
(pages 120–121)

9 **Good Mornings**
(pages 110–111)

Other targeted workouts

Upper-Abdominal Workout
Strengthens and defines your upper abs.
· Plank-Up (pages 78–79)
· T-Stabilization (pages 84–85)
· Mountain Climber (pages 92–93)
· Sit-Up (pages 100–101)
· One-Armed Sit-Up (pages 102–103)
· Crunch (pages 104–105)
· V-Up (pages 106–107)
· Penguin Crunch (pages 114–115)
· Wood Chop with Fitness Ball
  (pages 116–117)
· Fitness Ball Seated Russian Twist
  (pages 118–119)

Lower-Abdominal Workout
Strengthens and defines your lower abs.
· Side Plank (pages 80–81)
· Fire Hydrant In-Out (pages 82–83)
· T-Stabilization (pages 84–85)

· Hip Crossover (pages 98–99)
· Hip Raise (pages 96–97)
· Reverse Crunch (pages 108–109)
· Good Mornings (pages 110–111)
· Leg Raise (pages 120–121)
· Superman (pages 122–123)
· Fitness Ball Russian Twist
  (pages 112–113)

Global Workout
Incorporates core stabilization and core
strengthening for maximum efficiency.
· Side Plank (pages 80–81)
· T-Stabilization (pages 84–85)
· Fitness Ball Rollout (pages 88–89)
· Fitness Ball Hyperextension
  (pages 90–91)
· Hip Crossover (pages 98–99)
· One-Armed Sit-Up (pages 102–103)
· V-Up (pages 106–107)

· Reverse Crunch (pages 108–109)
· Penguin Crunch (pages 114–115)
· Leg Raises (pages 120–121)

Warrior Workout
Challenges the diehard who wants
to maximize core stability, strength,
athleticism, and ab definition.
· Plank-Up (pages 78–79)
· T-Stabilization (pages 84–85)
· Fitness Ball Atomic Push-Up
  (pages 86–87)
· Body-Weight Squat (pages 94–95)
· One-Armed Sit-Up (pages 102–103)
· V-Up (pages 106–107)
· Penguin Crunch (pages 114–115)
· Fitness Ball Seated Russian Twist
  (pages 118–119)
· Leg Raise (pages 120–121)
· Superman (pages 122–123)

Athlete's Workout

This workout gears up your core for the rotational performance that many sports demand.

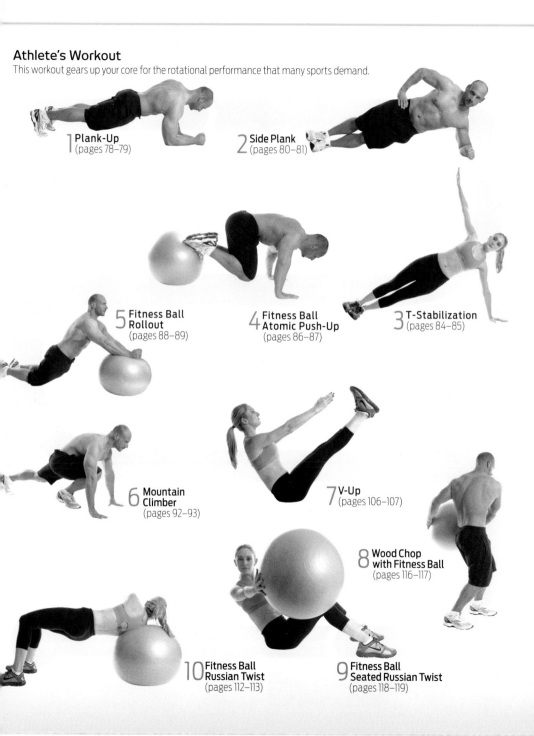

1 Plank-Up
(pages 78–79)

2 Side Plank
(pages 80–81)

3 T-Stabilization
(pages 84–85)

4 Fitness Ball
Atomic Push-Up
(pages 86–87)

5 Fitness Ball
Rollout
(pages 88–89)

6 Mountain
Climber
(pages 92–93)

7 V-Up
(pages 106–107)

8 Wood Chop
with Fitness Ball
(pages 116–117)

9 Fitness Ball
Seated Russian Twist
(pages 118–119)

10 Fitness Ball
Russian Twist
(pages 112–113)

About the Author

Hollis Lance Liebman has been a fitness magazine editor, national bodybuilding champion, and author. He is a published physique photographer and has served as a bodybuilding and fitness competition judge. Currently a Los Angeles resident, Hollis has worked with some of Hollywood's elite, earning rave reviews. Visit his Web site, www.holliswashere.com, for fitness tips and complete training programs.

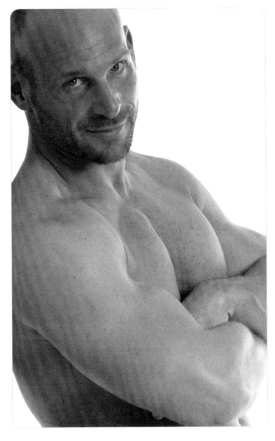

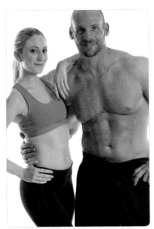

Core model Cori D. Cohen is a registered dietitian and healthy lifestyle coach based in New York City. She provides private nutrition counseling to a diverse clientele, in addition to working with residents at a nursing and rehabilitation center. Ms. Cohen has degrees from the University of Delaware, Fashion Institute of Technology, CUNY Queens College, and LIU C.W. Post. She is currently featured as a columnist for the *Queens Courier*, where she provides readers with valuable nutrition advice.

ANATOMY OF FITNESS™

Pilates

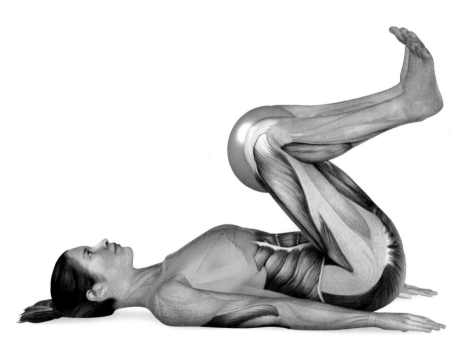

Created by Moseley Road Inc.
Editorial director: Lisa Purcell
Art director: Brian MacMullen
Cover and internals designer: Sam Grimmer
Photographer: Jonathan Conklin Photography, Inc.
Author: Isabel Eisen
Model: Brooke Marrone
Illustrator: Hector Aiza/3DLabz
Inset illustrations: Linda Bucklin/Shutterstock.com,
page 133 Venus Angel/Shutterstock.com
Prepress: Graphic Print Group

Contents

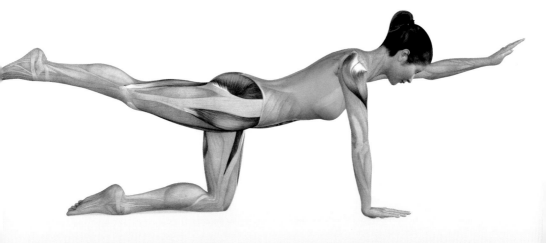

Pilates: Fitness for Life

Pilates is a rewarding and invigorating exercise program. It not only accomplishes wonders for a wide range of people, but it can also be practiced anytime and anywhere.

The Pilates method is a balanced, safe, and effective approach to fitness conditioning. Whether your goals involve work or everyday activities, sports performance, injury prevention, or "just" the need for better overall health, as a student of Pilates you'll experience improvement in physical stability, strength, and flexibility. Pilates helps to keep your body and mind aligned throughout your lifetime. With regular practice, you'll look great and feel amazing.

With step-by-step instructions, photos, and anatomical illustrations, this book offers a comprehensive guide to practicing Pilates at home. We'll look at the origins of Pilates, talk about the essential principles of the system, introduce you to some very useful terms, and talk about your "powerhouse," that core of muscles that is the central focus of all Pilates work.

History of Pilates

Joseph Pilates developed the Pilates system (originally called Contrology), during the early part of the twentieth century in Germany, where he was born, and then in New York City, where he taught from 1926 to 1966. Although he was a fragile child, he eventually became an accomplished gymnast, body builder, and physical trainer, and he designed rehabilitation equipment and exercises for bedridden prisoners of war during World War II. Inspired as he was by philosophies embodied in yoga, Zen Buddhism, Chinese martial arts, and the ancient Greek ideal of the perfect integrated human, as well as his studies of anatomy, Joseph Pilates developed a method of exercising grounded in the connection between body and mind.

Pilates built his method on six primary principles: centering, control, flow, breath, precision, and concentration (see "The Pilates Principles," pages 134–135). The discipline of Pilates, then as now, consists of exercises that flow into one another at a controlled pace, that progress from smaller to larger movements, from lying on a mat to standing on it—always with an awareness of the correct alignment of the body in space.

A new tradition

Dancers and elite athletes have always been faithful students of the Pilates method. In the 1980s, however, the Pilates method of training exploded in popularity as developments in exercise science moved quite beautifully into alignment with Joseph Pilates' methodology. The "pain makes gain" approach to exercising was re-evaluated, did a flip, and landed on its feet facing a new direction. Qualitative processes were now considered at least as important as the once all-important quantitative results.

Joseph Pilates' Contrology has long held a respected place among physical therapists and other professionals who work in the healthcare field. Pilates helps the healthy to remain healthy, strong, supple, and physically alert. Targeted programs focus on athletic, post-rehabilitation, and pre- and postnatal conditioning, as well as helping to improve lower-back-pain problems and aging issues.

Exercise and energy

Your goal is to have enough energy to perform an intense, dynamic, and invigorating fitness workout, so make sure that you have sufficient fuel for your body and mind to work in harmony—creating and maintaining a happy, vitalized, and healthy you.

Practitioners of Pilates usually find that they have better posture, and feel more "aligned and together," when they leave the mat to tackle the multitude of activities that compose their daily lives. Pilates exercise also raises an awareness of the impact of deep lateral breathing, which in turn generates more efficient movement, better blood circulation and more energy, stamina, and vigor.

Remember: the quality of your movement while exercising is always more important than any quantitative striving you do along the way. Let's take a look at the Pilates Principles to understand why.

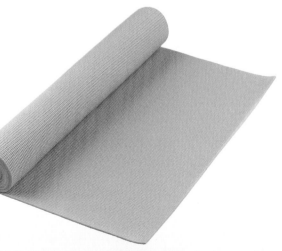

The Pilates Principles

Centering, control, flow, breath, precision, and concentration are often invoked as the foundations of the Pilates approach to fitness, or the Pilates Principles.

To get the most from your Pilates workout, you need to master these main principles.

Centering

Movement radiates from the "powerhouse" of strong muscles around your lumbar spine—between the bottom of the ribs and the line across the hips—into your arms and legs. *Centering* means bringing your awareness to this powerhouse and performing movements from this central core: your belly, lower back, hips, and buttocks. The powerhouse encompasses the rectus abdominis, obliquus internus and externus, multifidus spinae, and transversus abdominis, along with the pelvic floor muscles, diaphragm, gluteal muscles, and psoas. These muscles stabilize the lower limbs. Around your shoulder girdle, there's another strong group of muscles that stabilizes the upper body and limbs. These muscles include the lower trapezius, serratus anterior, latissimus dorsi, pectoralis major and minor, and deep neck flexors.

Control

In Pilates, *control* is defined as an awareness of the what, where, why, when, and how of an exercise. Controlled exercising develops good posture, strength, stamina, flexibility, and ease of movement, and is a tool for re-establishing our physical equilibrium when we need to find it again as, for example, after an injury. Those few Pilates exercises that use momentum, such as rolling and jumping exercises, are still performed with complete control. When you control your movement, you must be strong and flexible enough to allow your movement and breath to flow, grow, and lengthen.

Flow

Although it sounds self-evident that movement should move, it can become all too easy to neglect flow by "forgetting" to breathe, or breathing in a shallow, impractical way. Pilates emphasizes lengthening the body, stretching away from the center, while keeping the body compact and strong. *Flow* relates to the quality of your movement, too. Challenge yourself to keep the flow of movement

Visual imaging

Visual imaging is often used as a basic tool in Pilates training. These images are metaphors that engage both mind and body, helping us to use our muscles correctly. Some examples of these images are: zipping up your front, plugging your shoulders down your back, moving from your hip creases, and elongating your spine like a dart in space.

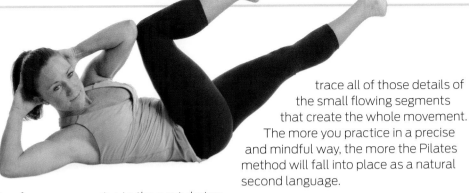

trace all of those details of the small flowing segments that create the whole movement. The more you practice in a precise and mindful way, the more the Pilates method will fall into place as a natural second language.

going from one exercise to the next during the transitions. Move smoothly from the end position of one exercise into the next one's starting position. How do you know if you're in "flow"? If you feel awkward while moving, or feel any strain, then try again.

Breath

In the Pilates system, you breathe in deeply through your nose and expand your lower ribcage out through your sides (laterally) and fully into your back. When you exhale through your mouth, your ribcage relaxes downward compactly, as if you were snapping together two sides of a tightly fitting shirt. Your spine should remain flexible, though with a sensation of lengthening all the time. Exhalation usually happens during the more arduous parts of an exercise, and inhalation on the preparation and return parts. Never hold your *breath* while exercising because you're so busy focusing on the exercise sequence.

Precision

While performing exercises, *precision* makes it possible to move forward rapidly and develop an intuitive understanding of each one's purpose. Pilates is not all about positioning, but it *is* about being able to

Concentration

In Pilates, *concentration* involves the vital mind/body connection. It's not enough to just execute a movement; you have to focus on what you're doing. You can create an image of yourself performing an exercise correctly, in proper alignment. You can build up a rhythm of sensing—with as much clarity as possible—the balanced muscular pathway that's going to carry that movement to completion in a strong yet melodious flow. This type of body and mind-intertwined dialogue demands concentration.

Positioning

At the beginning of most Pilates exercises, you will find yourself in one of two positions: *neutral position*, in which the natural curve of your spine is maintained, or *imprinted position*, in which the lumbar spine can be lengthened. The neutral position is used when you lie on your back in a supine position with one or both feet on your mat. The imprinted position provides extra support for your lumbar; when imprinting, or "pressing the navel to the spine," the muscles of your lower back are both lengthened and strengthened and your abdominal wall is flattened.

Pilates at Home

An excellent place to start your study of Pilates is in your home. Matwork practice at home can accommodate any physical or time constraints that you may have.

With mindful practice, you can safely train without an instructor looking over your shoulder, because you'll mainly be lying on your back in a supine position or on your stomach in a prone position. What's more, with at-home practice you compete only with yourself, measuring progress against where you've come from—and where you want to go.

Your space

Your workout area need not be much larger than your Pilates mat. It should be uncluttered so that you can concentrate on the body-mind connection without being distracted, and clean so that you feel comfortable being near the floor. A nearby shelf or closet is useful for storing equipment, and a large mirror and/or anatomical posters of the human skeleton and the major muscles of the back and front might make interesting additions to your space.

What to wear

Any comfortable exercise clothes that allow you to have full range of motion should be fine. Just be aware that too much free-flowing fabric can hamper your practice; your wardrobe should be streamlined to your body shape so that you don't have to fidget and readjust your clothes after every movement.

Equipment

You actually have just about all the essentials to start practicing Pilates right now, today. You have your body, your intelligence, and your ability to use mindful images to affect your movement patterns. That's quite a lot already, isn't it?

Joseph Pilates believed that his exercises could be performed either on the floor or on a mat. The average Pilates mat is ½ inch/1.25 cm thick, supplies padding from the floor for movements like the rolling exercises, and should be made of foam firm enough to support balance exercises. If no mat is at hand, you can work on a carpet or use a blanket or towel.

Small equipment, such as the Pilates ring, can easily be incorporated into a home practice, unlike some of the bigger equipment found in many Pilates studios.

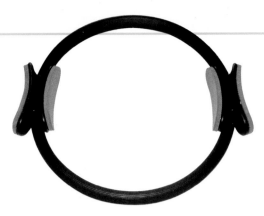

Making time for Pilates

Joseph Pilates suggested starting out by performing a few exercises in sequential order for just 10 minutes a day, four days a week, for at least three months. His belief—which still rings true today—was that the results should motivate us to increase the number of exercises performed during each session. This makes sense: the obvious rewards and benefits of the Pilates method will increase your desire to do more—and do it more often.

Set a realistic goal for yourself and commit to following your training schedule for three months, as Joseph Pilates suggested. After this period of time you'll have enough perspective to re-evaluate your regime and create a new set of goals for the next three-month period.

The small Pilates ball

Small pieces of equipment can add resistance, variety, and challenges to your home training. The small Pilates exercise ball imparts immediate extra awareness of core stability to just about any exercise. When grasped between the knees, it adds a new dimension to your exercise, helping to engage the hard-to-tone muscles of the inner thighs. If you don't have a Pilates ball, any small ball or even as cushion clasped between your knees or thighs will work.

And remember—you shouldn't blow a Pilates ball up all the way; instead, there should be a little give on the surface.

How to use this book

This book takes you through a sequence of 25 mat exercises that will give you a total-body workout, engaging your core, back, legs, and arms. First read the descriptive content about an exercise, and then refer to the photos and anatomical illustrations before you move into action. On each exercise page you'll find a short introduction to the exercise, step-by-step instructions explaining how to do it, some tips on how to perform it, and anatomical illustrations that show you just what muscles you are engaging.

Start by working through as many as you can, with the goal to build up your strength until you can perform all 25 in a smooth, uninterrupted flow.

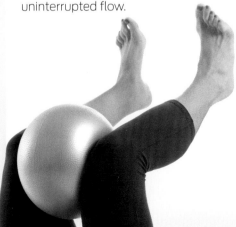

 DVD section 2: Chapter 1

Pointing Dog

Pointing Dog, also know as Four-Point Challenge or Pointer, targets your abdominal muscles, buttocks, hamstrings, and lumbar spine. This exercise strengthens your lower back and the fronts of your thighs, and it is one of those "easier" exercises that challenges your balance too.

1 Start on all fours, with your back in a neutral position, hands shoulder-width apart and fingertips facing forward. Place your wrists directly below your shoulders. Your thighs should form a straight line from hip joints to knees.

2 With control, extend one leg directly behind you while extending the opposite arm in front of you so that your extended arm and leg stretch in opposition to each other.

3 Hold this strong level position for 2 to 5 seconds. Return to the starting position. Repeat on the opposite side.

4 Repeat, completing a total of 10 repetitions (5 per side). Try working up to 3 sets of 10.

Correct form
· Keep your abdominals fully engaged, navel pressing toward your spine.
· Press your shoulder blades firmly down your back.

Avoid
· Changing the level of your pelvis.
· Arching your neck.

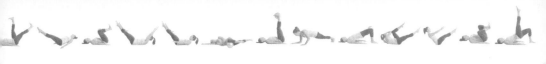

Diary of practice

	Date	Repetitions	Comment
Week 1			
Week 2			
Week 3			
Week 4			

Annotation Key
* indicates deep muscles

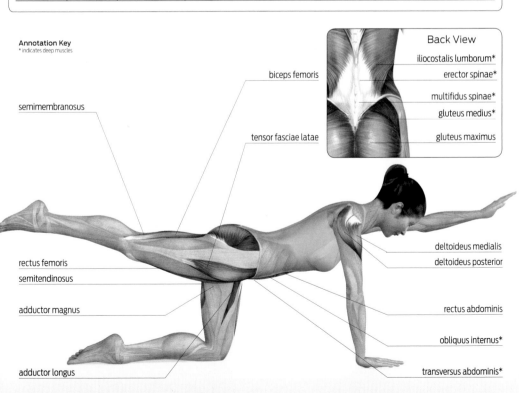

Back View

iliocostalis lumborum*
erector spinae*
multifidus spinae*
gluteus medius*
gluteus maximus

biceps femoris

semimembranosus

tensor fasciae latae

rectus femoris

semitendinosus

adductor magnus

adductor longus

deltoideus medialis
deltoideus posterior

rectus abdominis

obliquus internus*

transversus abdominis*

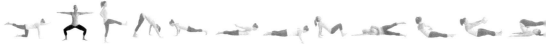

 DVD section 2: Chapter 2

Wide-Legged Plié

Wide-Legged Plié, borrowed from ballet training, targets your inner thighs and buttocks, helping you to attain lean and toned legs. Pliés also strengthen your back muscles and abdominals and increase mobility in your hips.

1 Stand with your feet 2 to 3 feet apart, turned out from your hips. Your heels should be rotated forward, and your knees aligned directly over your feet.

2 Maintain a neutral pelvis as you press your navel toward your spine, using your abdominals to lift your arms out to the sides at shoulder height—and within your peripheral vision.

3 Keeping your torso erect, slowly bend your knees, maintaining rotation in your legs.

4 Return to standing position, engaging your buttocks strongly, especially as you reach the top.

5 Repeat 10 to 12 times.

Correct form
· Keep your pelvis neutral and level.
· Lengthen your shoulders down your back.
· Keep your weight slightly shifted toward your heels during the exercise to prevent your knees and feet from rolling in.

Avoid
· Allowing your knees to extend past your toes.
· Altering the position of your hips.
· Rotating your leg from the knees, instead of from the hips.
· Locking your knees.

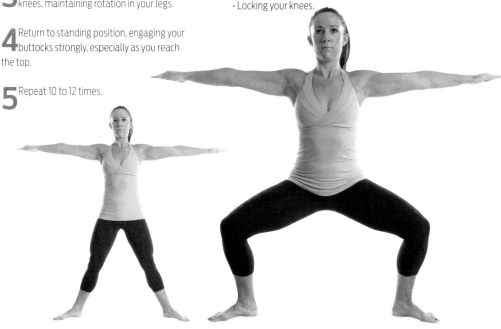

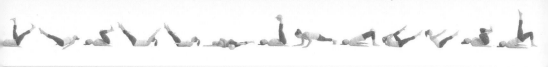

Diary of practice

	Date	Repetitions	Comment
Week 1			
Week 2			
Week 3			
Week 4			

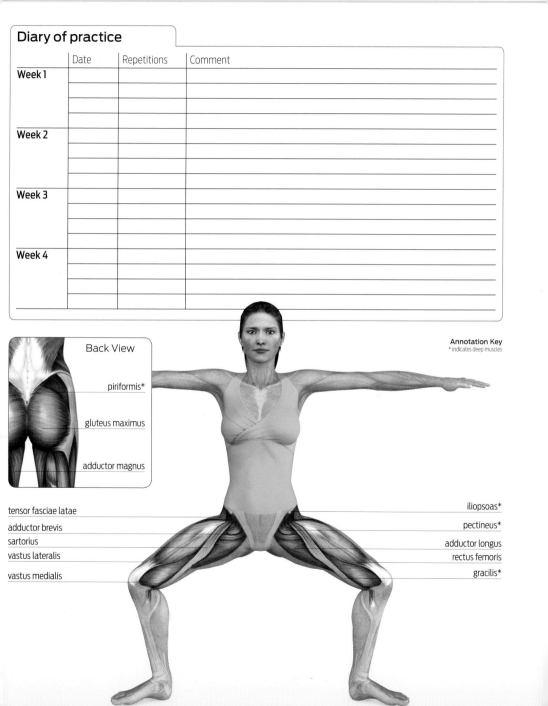

Back View

piriformis*

gluteus maximus

adductor magnus

Annotation Key
* indicates deep muscles

tensor fasciae latae

adductor brevis

sartorius

vastus lateralis

vastus medialis

iliopsoas*

pectineus*

adductor longus

rectus femoris

gracilis*

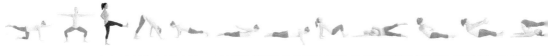

 DVD section 2: Chapter 3

Standing Leg Extension

Standing Leg Extension looks deceptively simple, but performing it correctly takes concentration. This exercise strengthens your quadriceps, that large group of muscles in the front of your thigh, and tones your abdominals and buttocks. It works your balance too. While standing on one leg, it helps to focus your eyes on a spot in front of you.

1 Stand with your legs together. Engage your abdominal muscles to stabilize your shoulders and your spine.

2 Glide your shoulders down your back to open your chest. Place your hands on your hips.

3 Bend one knee and lift your leg until your thigh is parallel to the mat, ankle flexed.

4 Keeping your ankle flexed, straighten your leg in front of you. Extend the leg only to a height at which you can continue to work the entire leg from the hip joint—while keeping your hips level.

5 Slowly bend your knee, returning it to a 90-degree angle. Complete 10 repetitions and then switch sides and repeat. Try to increase to 2 sets of 10 as you build up your strength and stamina.

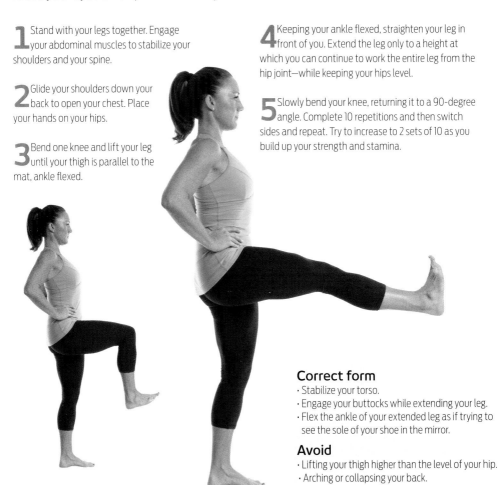

Correct form
· Stabilize your torso.
· Engage your buttocks while extending your leg.
· Flex the ankle of your extended leg as if trying to see the sole of your shoe in the mirror.

Avoid
· Lifting your thigh higher than the level of your hip.
· Arching or collapsing your back.

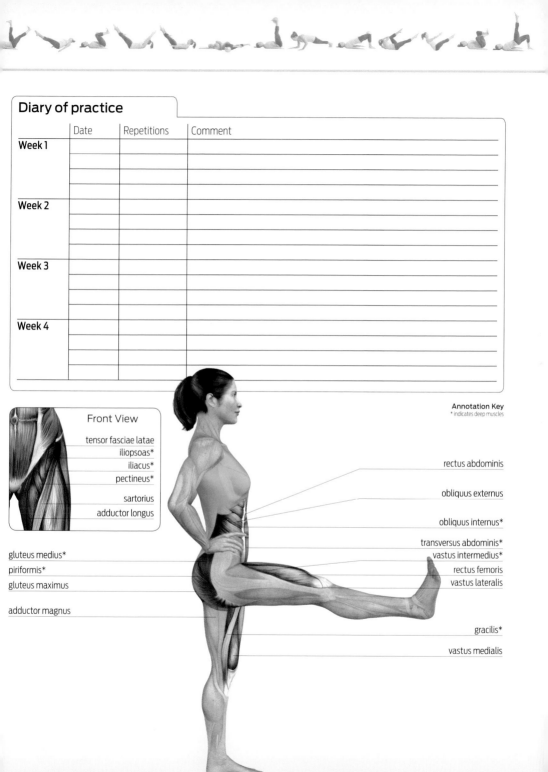

Diary of practice

	Date	Repetitions	Comment
Week 1			
Week 2			
Week 3			
Week 4			

Annotation Key
* indicates deep muscles

Front View

tensor fasciae latae
iliopsoas*
iliacus*
pectineus*
sartorius
adductor longus

gluteus medius*
piriformis*
gluteus maximus

adductor magnus

rectus abdominis

obliquus externus

obliquus internus*

transversus abdominis*
vastus intermedius*
rectus femoris
vastus lateralis

gracilis*

vastus medialis

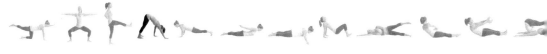

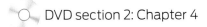

○ DVD section 2: Chapter 4

Monkey Walk

Monkey Walk is a good gauge of your fitness level—it's a full-body stretch that really tests the limits of your flexibility. Beginners may find it difficult to keep their knees and back straight, but with practice, you can learn to smoothly move from one phase of the exercise to the next.

1 From a standing, parallel position—and starting from the top of your head—peel your spine downward toward the floor.

2 Slowly "walk" your hands out to a plank position with your wrists directly under your shoulders. Keep your body parallel to the floor, legs hip-width apart, navel pressing toward your spine and shoulders pressing down your back.

3 Pop your hips toward the ceiling and push your weight back to your heels. Your body should be in the shape of an upside-down V. Hold for a few seconds before slowly walking your hands back toward your legs.

4 Complete 5 repetitions.

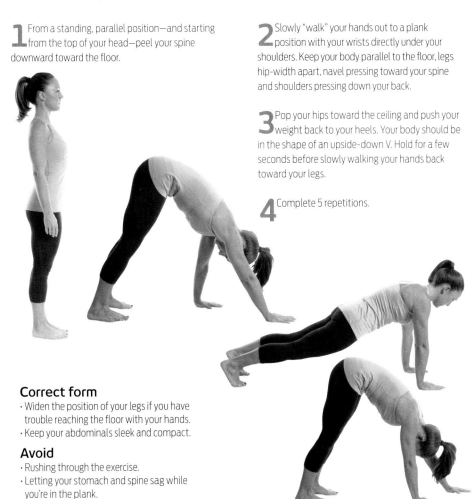

Correct form
· Widen the position of your legs if you have trouble reaching the floor with your hands.
· Keep your abdominals sleek and compact.

Avoid
· Rushing through the exercise.
· Letting your stomach and spine sag while you're in the plank.

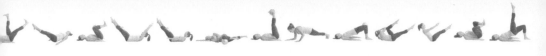

Diary of practice

	Date	Repetitions	Comment
Week 1			
Week 2			
Week 3			
Week 4			

Annotation Key
* indicates deep muscles

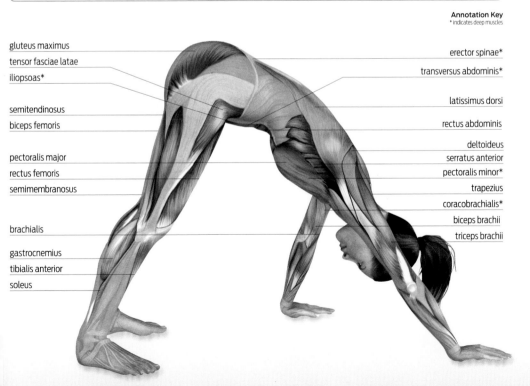

gluteus maximus
tensor fasciae latae
iliopsoas*

semitendinosus
biceps femoris

pectoralis major
rectus femoris
semimembranosus

brachialis

gastrocnemius
tibialis anterior
soleus

erector spinae*
transversus abdominis*

latissimus dorsi
rectus abdominis

deltoideus
serratus anterior
pectoralis minor*
trapezius
coracobrachialis*
biceps brachii
triceps brachii

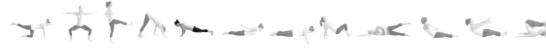

Push-Up

The Push-Up, also known as a Press-Up, is a well-known calisthenics exercise performed everywhere: school gyms, Pilates and judo studios, and military boot camps too. The reason for this is its effectiveness—it's a basic exercise that really works your chest, shoulders, back, and core.

1 Start on your hands and knees, with your hands slightly wider apart than shoulder-width. Extend your legs backward to come into a high plank position.

2 With control, slowly lower the full length of your body toward the mat, bending your elbows. Stop when your elbows are at 90 degrees.

3 Straighten your elbows and return to your plank position.

4 Start with 1 set of 8 repetitions. Try to work up to 3 sets of 12 repetitions.

Correct form
· Keep your shoulders pressing down your back.
· Imagine a straight line running from the top of your head to your heels.

Avoid
· Compromising the neutral alignment of your pelvis and spine.

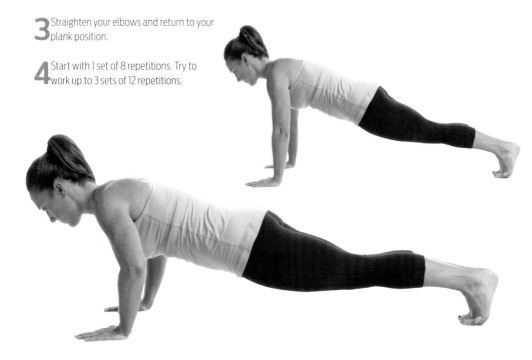

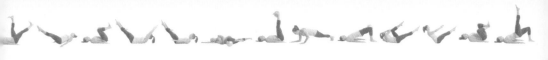

Diary of practice

	Date	Repetitions	Comment
Week 1			
Week 2			
Week 3			
Week 4			

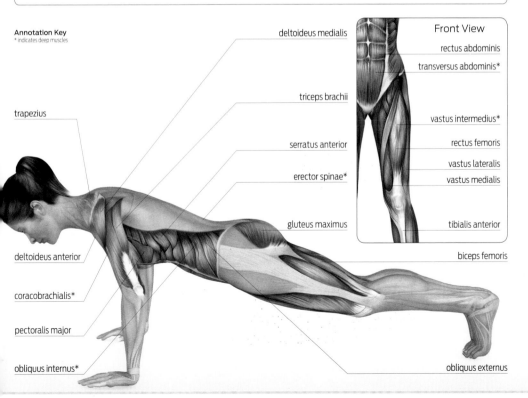

Annotation Key
* indicates deep muscles

deltoideus medialis

triceps brachii

trapezius

serratus anterior

erector spinae*

gluteus maximus

deltoideus anterior

coracobrachialis*

pectoralis major

obliquus internus*

Front View

rectus abdominis

transversus abdominis*

vastus intermedius*

rectus femoris

vastus lateralis

vastus medialis

tibialis anterior

biceps femoris

obliquus externus

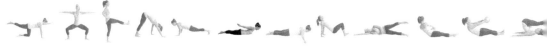

Breast Stroke

Breast Stroke adds another level of challenge to the classic Pilates Swimming exercise. It's a great stretcher and strengthener for your lower back.

1 Lie on your stomach with your legs extended behind you and feet pointed. Keeping your core stabilized, engage your abdominals. Bend your arms, holding your hands palms down, and raise them a few inches off the mat.

2 As if swimming the breast stroke, lift your upper chest off the mat as you bring your arms out to your sides and then behind you.

3 Bend your elbows close to your chest, and then extend your arms forward to return to the starting position.

4 Complete the entire sequence for 10 repetitions.

Correct form
· Keep your abdominals engaged throughout the exercise.

Avoid
· Rushing through the movement—imagine the resistance of water as you move.
· Lifting your feet off the mat.
· Hunching your shoulders to your ears.

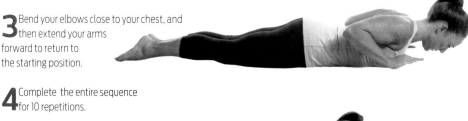

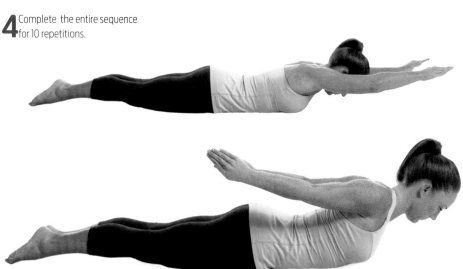

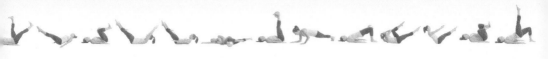

Diary of practice

	Date	Repetitions	Comment
Week 1			
Week 2			
Week 3			
Week 4			

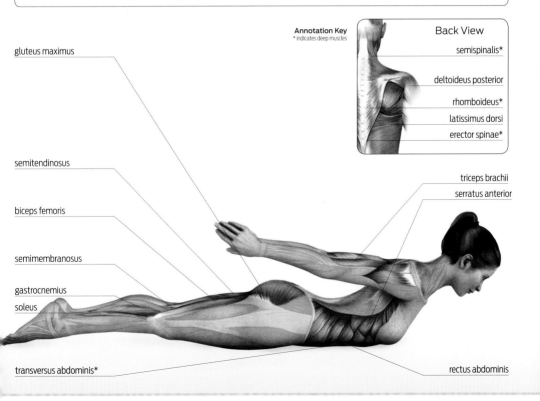

Annotation Key
* indicates deep muscles

Back View

semispinalis*

deltoideus posterior

rhomboideus*

latissimus dorsi

erector spinae*

gluteus maximus

semitendinosus

biceps femoris

semimembranosus

gastrocnemius

soleus

transversus abdominis*

triceps brachii

serratus anterior

rectus abdominis

Back Burner

In addition to strengthening your lower back, Back Burner strengthens all of your abdominal muscles. You'll build a sound core and improve your posture in the process.

1 Lie on your stomach with your arms extended in front of you. Your legs should be weighted into the mat with feet pointed. Press your navel to your spine, and your shoulders down your back.

2 Lift your extended arms off the mat and pulse them up and down 10 to 15 times.

3 Reposition your arms so that they are at 10:00 and 2:00 on an imaginary clock. Complete 10 to 15 more pulses from this position.

4 Keeping your shoulders down, move your arms to 3:00 and 9:00 position, and perform 10 to 15 more pulses.

5 Bring both arms behind you, angled slightly with palms inward, and pulse 10 to 15 times, with the action originating from your shoulders. Work up to 10 repetitions.

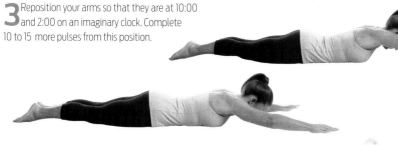

Correct form
· Keep your abdominals strong and your hips stable.
· Look toward the mat to elongate your neck.
· Keep your torso and legs still throughout.
· Move your arms from under your shoulder blades.

Avoid
· Hunching your shoulders.
· Lifting your feet off the mat.

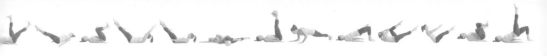

Diary of practice

	Date	Repetitions	Comment
Week 1			
Week 2			
Week 3			
Week 4			

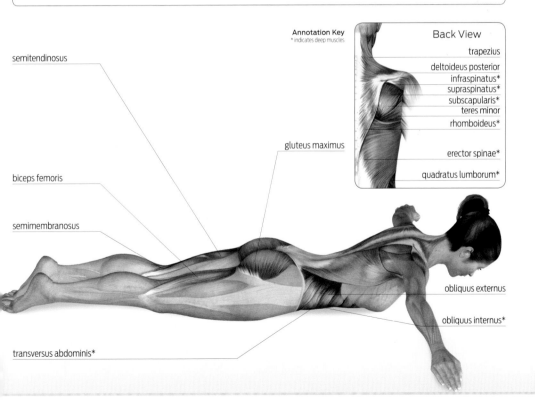

Annotation Key
* indicates deep muscles

semitendinosus

biceps femoris

semimembranosus

transversus abdominis*

gluteus maximus

obliquus externus

obliquus internus*

Back View

trapezius
deltoideus posterior
infraspinatus*
supraspinatus*
subscapularis*
teres minor
rhomboideus*

erector spinae*

quadratus lumborum*

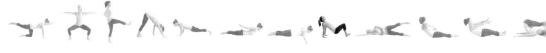

Triceps Dip

You'll really feel the effects of Triceps Dip on the backs of your arms when you do this exercise correctly. The Dip engages everything else too, due to the effort that's needed to keep your body in position. Balancing on your heels throughout the exercise pushes your body weight toward your upper body so that your triceps have to work harder to support you.

1 Sit on your mat with your knees bent. Your arms should be behind you with your elbows bent and the palms of your hands pressing into the mat, fingers facing forward. Straighten your arms as you lift your hips a few inches off the mat.

2 Shift your weight back toward your arms, and keeping your heels pressed firmly into the mat, lift your toes off the mat.

3 Bend your elbows, keeping your chest open and your gaze diagonally upward.

4 Keeping your chest open, use your arms to lift your body up again.

5 Perform 2 to 3 sets of 10 to 12 repetitions.

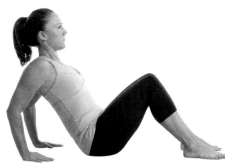

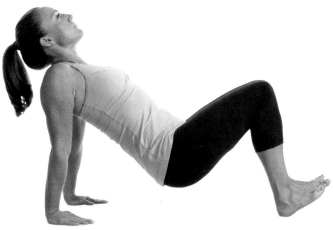

Correct form
· Keep your chest lifted and open.
· Hold your shoulders down.

Avoid
· Arching your back.
· Lifting your shoulders.
· Rushing through the exercise.

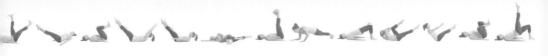

Diary of practice

	Date	Repetitions	Comment
Week 1			
Week 2			
Week 3			
Week 4			

Annotation Key
* indicates deep muscles

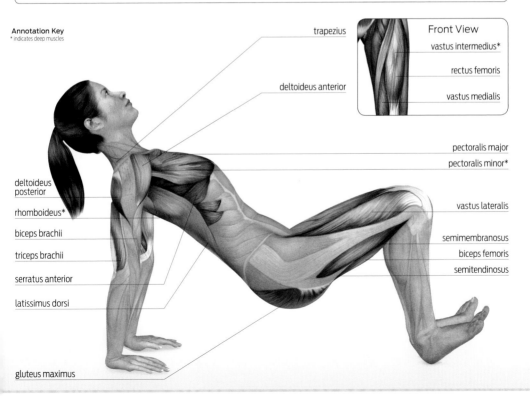

trapezius

deltoideus anterior

Front View

vastus intermedius*

rectus femoris

vastus medialis

pectoralis major
pectoralis minor*

deltoideus posterior

rhomboideus*

biceps brachii

triceps brachii

serratus anterior

latissimus dorsi

gluteus maximus

vastus lateralis

semimembranosus
biceps femoris
semitendinosus

Side Leg Series

Getting the most out of Side Leg Series means keeping your core muscles completely still while your lower body moves: challenging, but well worth it. Over time you should achieve toned thighs and a sleeker, tighter midsection.

1 Lie on your side with your legs extended forward at a 45-degree angle to your body. Straighten your bottom arm and bend the other so that your hand is on the mat in front of you. Press your navel toward your spine and align your hips on top of each other.

2 Lift your top leg and flex your foot. From your hip joint, slightly rotate your foot toward the mat and move your leg up and down 25 times.

3 Next, point your foot and lift your leg, and then flex your foot and lower your leg. Complete 25 repetitions.

4 Next, lift your top leg no higher than your hip and flex your foot. Maintaining a strong flexed foot, perform 50 pulses.

5 Repeat the entire series up to 5 times on each side.

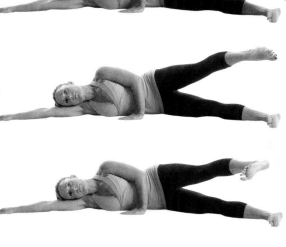

Correct form
- Keep your top leg directly above your bottom leg throughout.
- Keep your foot rotated toward the mat, whether flexed or pointed.

Avoid
- Moving your upper body or hips at any point in the exercise. Use your strong core to stabilize your upper body and "drive" the movement.
- Locking your knees.
- Losing the 45-degree angle of the legs during the exercise.

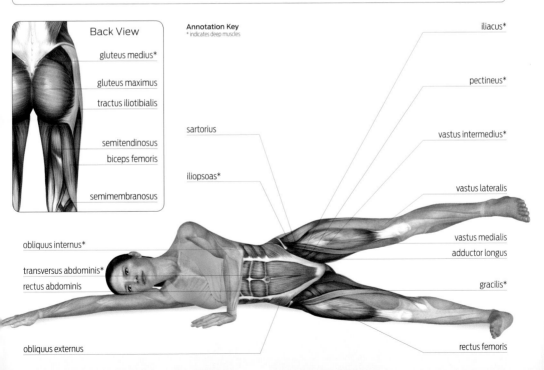

Diary of practice

	Date	Repetitions	Comment
Week 1			
Week 2			
Week 3			
Week 4			

Back View

gluteus medius*

gluteus maximus

tractus iliotibialis

semitendinosus

biceps femoris

semimembranosus

Annotation Key
* indicates deep muscles

sartorius

iliopsoas*

obliquus internus*

transversus abdominis*

rectus abdominis

obliquus externus

iliacus*

pectineus*

vastus intermedius*

vastus lateralis

vastus medialis

adductor longus

gracilis*

rectus femoris

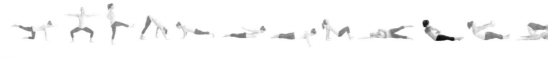

 DVD section 2: Chapter 10

Waistline Warrior

Waistline Warrior may look simple enough, but these small movements really challenge your oblique muscles.

1 Sit with your legs extended in front of you. With a Pilates ball between your hands, extend your arms forward. Imprint your pelvis, and curl slightly backward, so you're in a balanced position right behind your sit-bones in a shallow C-curve.

2 Keeping your abdominals tight and your legs firmly on the mat, squeeze your inner thighs and rotate your torso slightly to the right, bringing the ball with you.

3 Slowly return to center and then repeat on the other side.

4 Complete 10 repetitions, alternating sides.

Correct form
- Curl back only as far as you can maintain control of your abdominals and legs.
- Follow the ball with your gaze.
- Hold your arms in a slightly curved shape.

Avoid
- Lifting your legs off the ground.
- Rushing through the movement; your pace should be smooth, steady, and controlled.

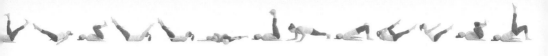

Diary of practice

	Date	Repetitions	Comment
Week 1			
Week 2			
Week 3			
Week 4			

Annotation Key
* indicates deep muscles

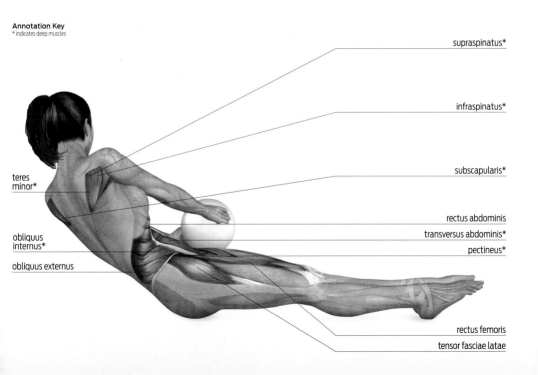

supraspinatus*

infraspinatus*

subscapularis*

rectus abdominis

transversus abdominis*

pectineus*

rectus femoris

tensor fasciae latae

teres minor*

obliquus internus*

obliquus externus

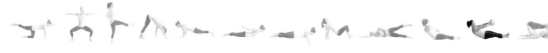

 DVD section 2: Chapter 11

Pilates Ball Roll-Up

Using a Pilates ball puts a new twist on the classic Pilates Roll-Up, which challenges your powerhouse muscles, flattens your abdominals, and strengthens your back. Let your breath guide you through the exercise, so that you use the same control rolling down as you do rolling up. Master this one and your abdominals and back will thank you.

1 Lie on the mat in a neutral position with your ankles strongly flexed. With the ball between your hands, glide your shoulder blades down your back as you lift your arms overhead, extended slightly above the mat behind you. Your shoulders and your rib cage should be pressed downward.

2 Press your navel to your spine, and, in sequence, roll up each vertebra from the mat, reaching your arms forward into the space above your legs. It helps to really press your heels into the mat.

3 Reverse the movement, keeping the ball at shoulder height and rolling into the mat vertebra by vertebra, controlling the urge to lift your shoulders and collapse your chest.

4 Complete 5 repetitions.

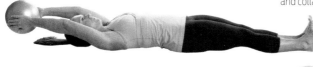

Correct form
· Keep your abdominals and rib cage strongly interlaced with your back.
· Keep pressing your legs and heels into the mat for stabilization.

Avoid
· Using shoulder or arm momentum to roll up or down.
· Bouncing or otherwise compromising the fluid steadiness of the movements.

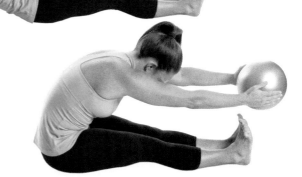

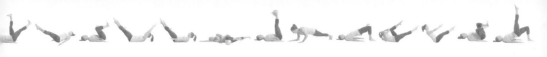

Diary of practice

	Date	Repetitions	Comment
Week 1			
Week 2			
Week 3			
Week 4			

Annotation Key
* indicates deep muscles

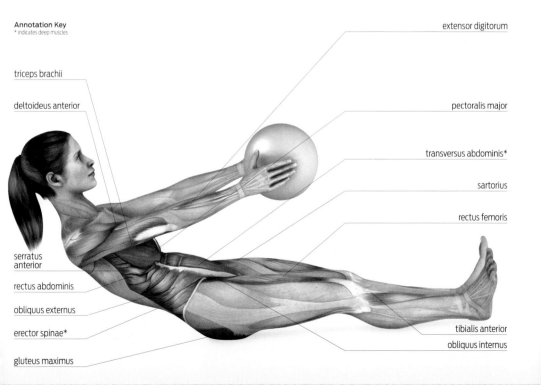

extensor digitorum

triceps brachii

deltoideus anterior

pectoralis major

transversus abdominis*

sartorius

rectus femoris

serratus anterior

rectus abdominis

obliquus externus

erector spinae*

tibialis anterior

obliquus internus

gluteus maximus

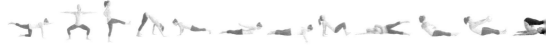

 DVD section 2: Chapter 12

Rollover

Another classic Pilates exercise, Rollover stretches and articulates
your spine and requires a high degree of core control and awareness.

1 Lie on your back with your arms along your
sides, palms down.

2 Lift your legs so that they form a
45-degree angle to the mat,
and flex your ankles. Engage
your abdominals, and
make sure that your
spine is stable on
the mat.

3 Press your arms into the mat to help stabilize
your torso and roll your extended legs back
toward your head, peeling your spine off the mat.

4 When you have reached the farthest position,
open your leg slightly, and with control, roll
sequentially through your spine to return your legs
to the starting position above your hips.

5 Repeat 4 to 6 times.

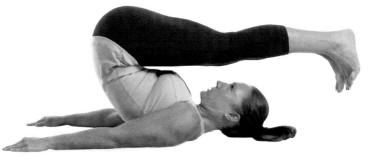

Correct form
· Stabilize your head and
  neck on the mat.
· Keep your abdominals
  strongly engaged
  throughout.

Avoid
· Rolling in a jerky manner:
  focus on fluidity of
  movement.

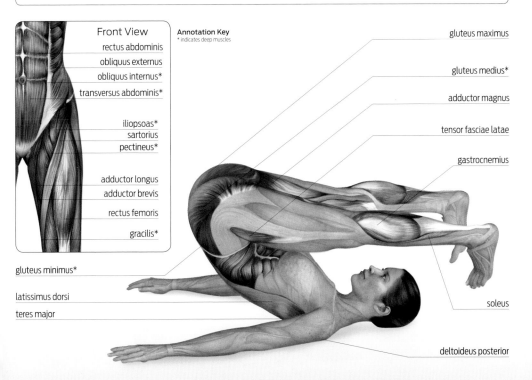

Diary of practice

	Date	Repetitions	Comment
Week 1			
Week 2			
Week 3			
Week 4			

Front View

rectus abdominis
obliquus externus
obliquus internus*
transversus abdominis*

iliopsoas*
sartorius
pectineus*

adductor longus
adductor brevis

rectus femoris

gracilis*

gluteus minimus*

latissimus dorsi

teres major

Annotation Key
* indicates deep muscles

gluteus maximus

gluteus medius*

adductor magnus

tensor fasciae latae

gastrocnemius

soleus

deltoideus posterior

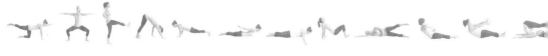

 DVD section 2: Chapter 13

Single Leg Drop

Single Leg Drop is an effective abdominal flattener. Try not to rush through the movement: it's essential that your upper body stay anchored to the ground as you lower and raise your leg—a movement driven by the strong, engaged muscles of your core.

1 Lie on your back with arms at your sides and legs extended straight upward. Flex your ankles.

2 Lower one of your legs from your hip socket, keeping your hips firmly fastened to your mat. Bring that leg directly over your hip socket again.

3 Repeat on the other side, working up to 20 repetitions (10 per leg).

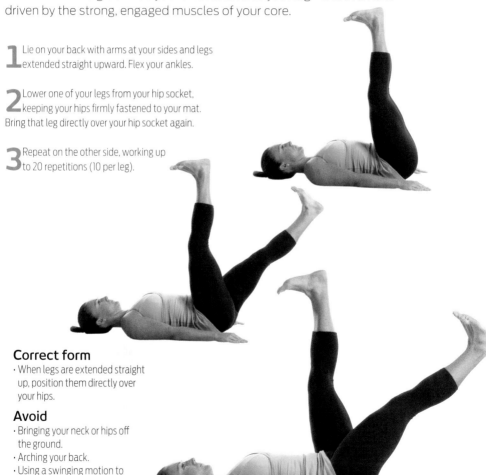

Correct form
· When legs are extended straight up, position them directly over your hips.

Avoid
· Bringing your neck or hips off the ground.
· Arching your back.
· Using a swinging motion to lower or raise your leg. Instead, maintain steady control throughout.

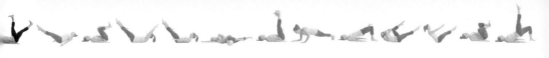

Diary of practice

	Date	Repetitions	Comment
Week 1			
Week 2			
Week 3			
Week 4			

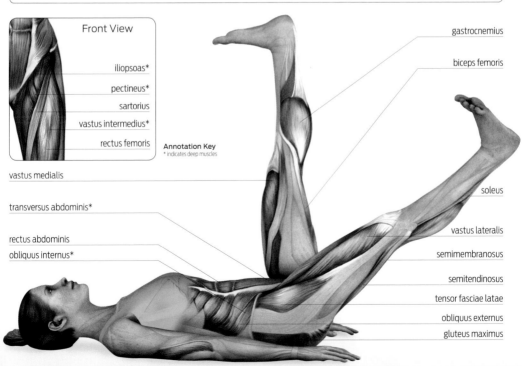

Front View

iliopsoas*
pectineus*
sartorius
vastus intermedius*
rectus femoris

Annotation Key
* indicates deep muscles

gastrocnemius

biceps femoris

vastus medialis

transversus abdominis*

rectus abdominis
obliquus internus*

soleus

vastus lateralis

semimembranosus

semitendinosus

tensor fasciae latae

obliquus externus

gluteus maximus

 DVD section 2: Chapter 14

Corkscrew

A classic Pilates mat exercise, Corkscrew strengthens all of the abdominal muscles, challenges torso stability, and stretches the spine. Be especially aware of stabilizing your shoulders and pelvis while you work.

1 Lie on your back with your arms along your sides, palms downward for stability. Lift your legs 90 degrees from the mat. Press your navel to your spine.

2 Tightly hug your legs together, and, moving them from your hip joints as if they were a single leg, "draw" small ovals in one direction. Repeat 5 times.

3 Keeping your spine firmly pressed into your mat, "draw" small ovals in the opposite direction. Repeat 5 times.

4 You can also perform this exercise with your knees slightly bent (though firmly pressed together) to prevent strain in your shoulders or hips.

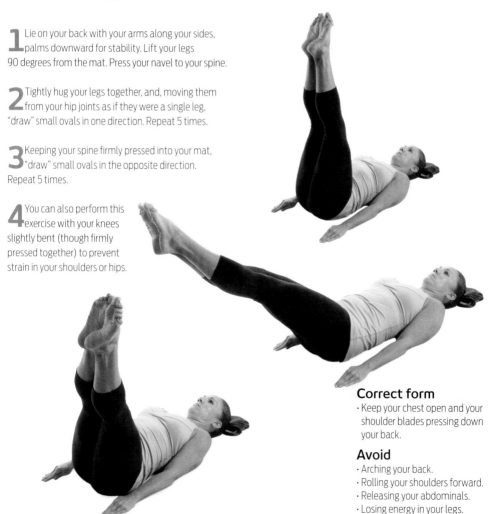

Correct form
· Keep your chest open and your shoulder blades pressing down your back.

Avoid
· Arching your back.
· Rolling your shoulders forward.
· Releasing your abdominals.
· Losing energy in your legs.

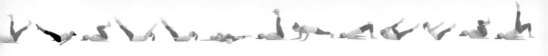

Diary of practice

	Date	Repetitions	Comment
Week 1			
Week 2			
Week 3			
Week 4			

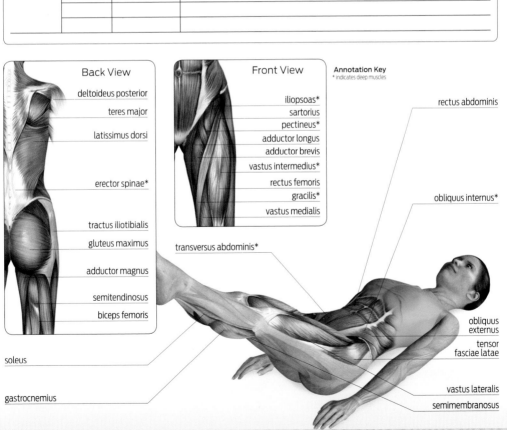

Back View

deltoideus posterior

teres major

latissimus dorsi

erector spinae*

tractus iliotibialis

gluteus maximus

adductor magnus

semitendinosus

biceps femoris

soleus

gastrocnemius

Front View

iliopsoas*

sartorius

pectineus*

adductor longus

adductor brevis

vastus intermedius*

rectus femoris

gracilis*

vastus medialis

transversus abdominis*

Annotation Key
* indicates deep muscles

rectus abdominis

obliquus internus*

obliquus externus

tensor fasciae latae

vastus lateralis

semimembranosus

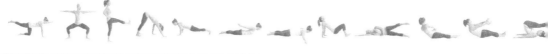

Pilates Ball Heel Tap

This version of Heel Tap improves your core stability and strength, enhancing your alignment and flattening your abdominals in the process. With the Pilates ball between your knees, your inner thighs get a great workout too.

1 Lie on your back with your arms along your sides, palms facedown, and the Pilates ball between your bent knees.

2 Keeping your upper body anchored on your mat, press your navel to your spine and dip your heels down toward your mat, hugging your inner thighs around the Pilates ball. Tap your heels to the mat.

3 Bring your legs back into your chest as you return to starting position.

4 Complete 10 repetitions.

Correct form
· Keep your abdominals strongly connected to your lower spine and your pelvis in imprint.

Avoid
· Arching your cervical or lumbar spine.

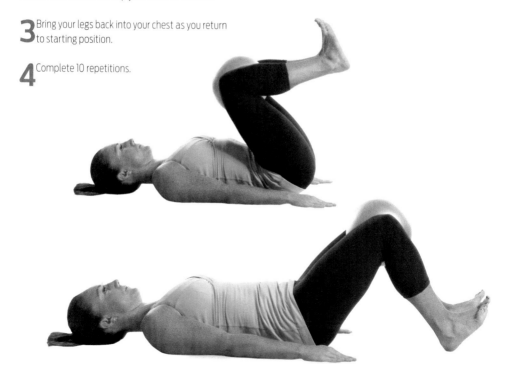

Diary of practice

	Date	Repetitions	Comment
Week 1			
Week 2			
Week 3			
Week 4			

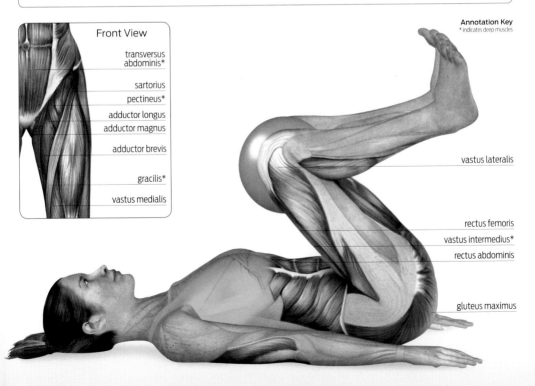

Front View

transversus abdominis*

sartorius

pectineus*

adductor longus

adductor magnus

adductor brevis

gracilis*

vastus medialis

Annotation Key
* indicates deep muscles

vastus lateralis

rectus femoris

vastus intermedius*

rectus abdominis

gluteus maximus

 DVD section 2: Chapter 16

Pilates Ball
Double Leg Stretch

Like so many Pilates exercises, Double Leg Stretch does an excellent job of toning your abdominals. The closer your extended arms and legs are to the floor, the harder it is to stabilize your torso—so start by lowering only to the level that you can control comfortably. Holding the Pilates ball between your legs targets the hard-to-reach inner-thigh muscles, making this an even more powerful workout for your whole body.

1 Lie on your back with your arms along your sides and your legs in tabletop position with the Pilates ball between your knees.

2 Engage your abdominals, and lift your head and shoulders off your mat, your arms extended toward your knees.

3 Using a strong core, extend your arms and legs in opposite directions.

4 Bring your arms and legs back to center, still pressing the ball between your knees.

5 Work up to 10 repetitions.

Correct form
· Keep the length of your spine supported on the mat in an imprint position.
· Maintain a stable pelvis.
· Engage your inner-thigh muscles to hold the ball in place.
· Gaze diagonally up and forward.

Avoid
· Losing control of your lower back as you extend your arms and legs.

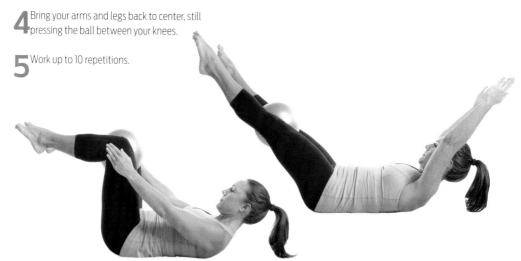

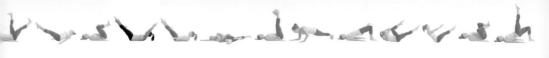

Diary of practice

	Date	Repetitions	Comment
Week 1			
Week 2			
Week 3			
Week 4			

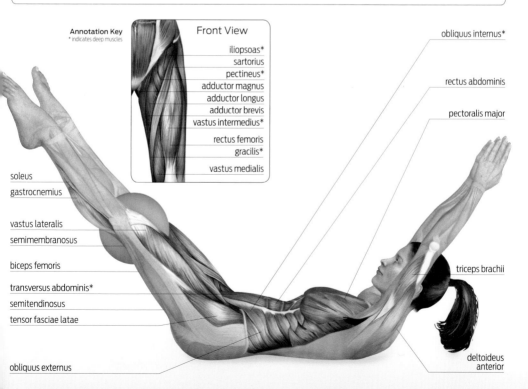

Annotation Key
* indicates deep muscles

Front View

iliopsoas*
sartorius
pectineus*
adductor magnus
adductor longus
adductor brevis
vastus intermedius*
rectus femoris
gracilis*
vastus medialis

obliquus internus*

rectus abdominis

pectoralis major

soleus

gastrocnemius

vastus lateralis

semimembranosus

biceps femoris

transversus abdominis*

semitendinosus

tensor fasciae latae

obliquus externus

triceps brachii

deltoideus
anterior

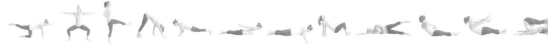

Pilates Ball Hundred

No Pilates session would be complete without the Hundred. Many value this exercise as a warm-up for the lungs, but it's also a serious abdominal toner in its own right. Holding the ball between your legs introduces lower-body resistance, ensuring that your thigh muscles reap great benefits as well.

1 Lie on your back, with your arms at your sides, your pelvis and spine in a neutral position, and your legs in tabletop with the Pilates ball between your knees.

2 Curl your head, neck, and shoulders a few inches off the mat, pressing your navel to your spine and imprinting your pelvis to the mat. Extend your arms so that they hover over your mat and extend your legs diagonally forward. Keep the ball stable between your knees and your feet pointed.

3 Move your arms in small pumping movements, breathing in for 5 counts and out for 5 counts. Complete 10 sets.

4 Bend your knees back to tabletop again, still holding the ball.

5 Lower your head, neck, and shoulders to your mat.

Correct form
· Press your navel down toward your spine and slide your rib cage down toward your pelvis.
· Maintain the imprint position of pelvis and spine throughout the exercise.
· Use your inner thighs to hold the ball in place.

Avoid
· Arching your lower back or neck.
· Lifting your shoulders.
· Locking your knees.

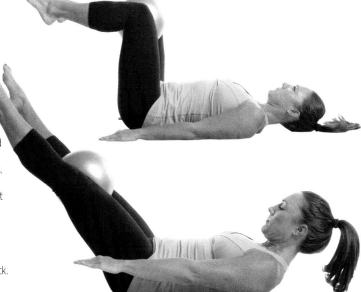

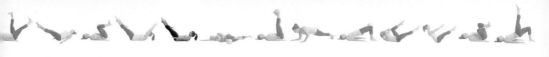

Diary of practice

	Date	Repetitions	Comment
Week 1			
Week 2			
Week 3			
Week 4			

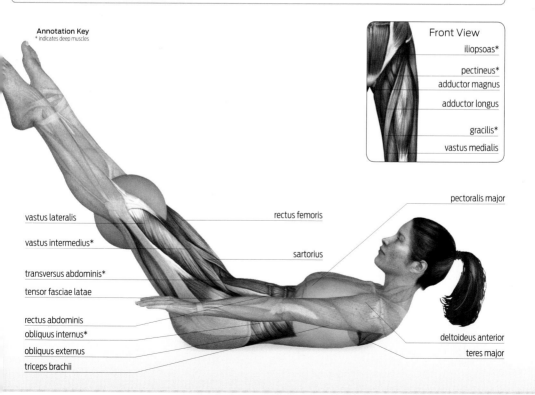

Annotation Key
* indicates deep muscles

Front View

iliopsoas*
pectineus*
adductor magnus
adductor longus
gracilis*
vastus medialis

pectoralis major

vastus lateralis

rectus femoris

vastus intermedius*

sartorius

transversus abdominis*

tensor fasciae latae

rectus abdominis

obliquus internus*

obliquus externus

deltoideus anterior

teres major

triceps brachii

 DVD section 2: Chapter 18

Pilates Ball Side-Lying Inner Thigh

Pilates Ball Side-Lying Inner Thigh strengthens and tones your hips, abdominals, and thighs. Keeping your hips and pelvis still as you pulse your leg is an exercise in core stability.

1 Lie on your side, with your hips and shoulders stacked. Extend your bottom arm and rest your head on it. Bend your top arm and place your palm on the mat in front of you, fingers pointing toward your head. Position your knee at a 90-degree angle to your hips, with the Pilates ball beneath it.

2 Lift your bottom leg off of the mat, keeping it strong and straight with the foot flexed parallel to your hips.

3 While your top leg stays at a 90-degree angle, move your bottom leg up and down 25 times.

4 Repeat on the other side.

Correct form
· Engage your top leg to keep the ball in place.
· Keep your abdominal muscles and rib cage strongly compact.

Avoid
· Tensing your shoulders and neck.

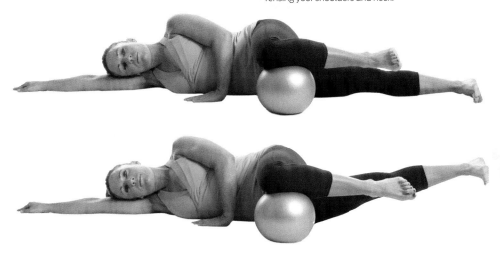

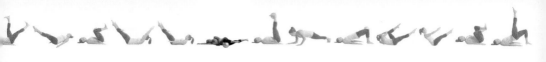

Diary of practice

	Date	Repetitions	Comment
Week 1			
Week 2			
Week 3			
Week 4			

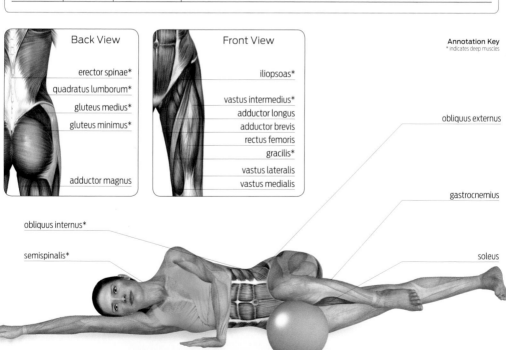

Back View

erector spinae*
quadratus lumborum*
gluteus medius*
gluteus minimus*

adductor magnus

Front View

iliopsoas*

vastus intermedius*
adductor longus
adductor brevis
rectus femoris
gracilis*

vastus lateralis
vastus medialis

Annotation Key
* indicates deep muscles

obliquus externus

gastrocnemius

obliquus internus*

semispinalis*

soleus

 DVD section 2: Chapter 19

Double Dip

Double Dip challenges your core muscles—the slower and more controlled your movement, the more quickly and noticeably your abdominals will benefit. Focus on keeping the Pilates ball still between your feet. Beyond engaging the muscles in your legs, this will help you to stay balanced, well-aligned, and in control throughout the movement.

1 Lie on your back, with your spine imprinted, your arms out along your sides, and your legs extended straight upward, holding the Pilates ball between your flexed feet.

2 Slowly and with control, lower your legs as far as you can while keeping your abdominals pulled in and your hips square on the mat. Keep the ball in place between your feet.

3 Just as slowly as you lowered them, raise your legs back to starting position.

4 Complete 5 repetitions.

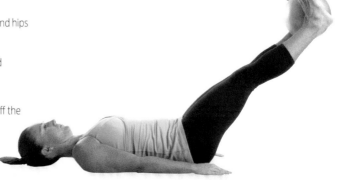

Correct form
· Keep your abdominals pulled in and hips flat on the ground.
· Move slowly and steadily.
· Focus on keeping the ball still and balanced between your feet.

Avoid
· Allowing your lower back to rise off the mat as you raise your legs.
· Rushing through the movement.
· Lifting your neck as you lower and raise your legs.

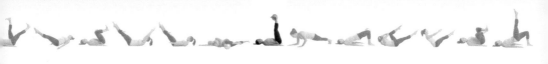

Diary of practice

	Date	Repetitions	Comment
Week 1			
Week 2			
Week 3			
Week 4			

Front View

rectus abdominis

iliopsoas*
sartorius
pectineus*
adductor longus
adductor magnus

vastus intermedius*

gracilis*
vastus medialis

vastus lateralis

rectus femoris

obliquus externus

Annotation Key
* indicates deep muscles

semimembranosus

biceps femoris

semitendinosus

transversus abdominis*

tensor fasciae latae

gluteus maximus

obliquus internus*

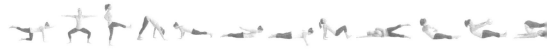

 DVD section 2: Chapter 20

Low-to-High Plank

If you want to tone your abdominals and arms, then Low-to-High Plank will do the job. Focus on keeping your abdominals fully engaged as you move from low to high and back again.

1 Start in Low Plank, with your weight evenly distributed on your elbows and the balls of your feet. Take a moment to stabilize your hips in this position and really engage your abdominals.

2 Reposition one arm and then the other so that your hands are on the mat in front of your shoulders, lifting your body into High Plank.

3 Return to Low Plank, repositioning one arm and then the other.

4 Start with 4 repetitions and work up to 12 on each arm.

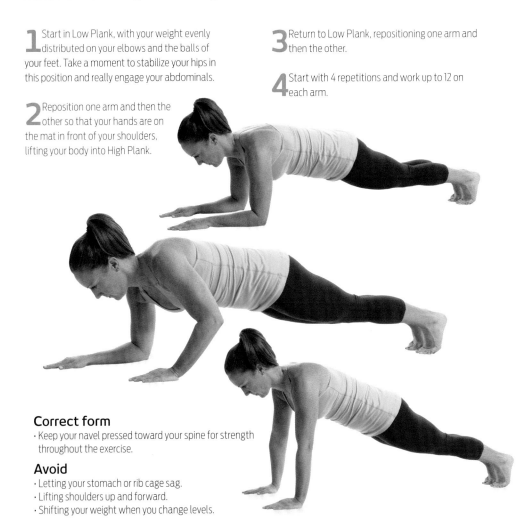

Correct form
· Keep your navel pressed toward your spine for strength throughout the exercise.

Avoid
· Letting your stomach or rib cage sag.
· Lifting shoulders up and forward.
· Shifting your weight when you change levels.

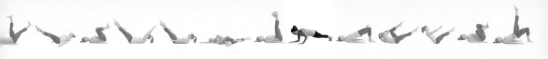

Diary of practice

	Date	Repetitions	Comment
Week 1			
Week 2			
Week 3			
Week 4			

Annotation Key
* indicates deep muscles

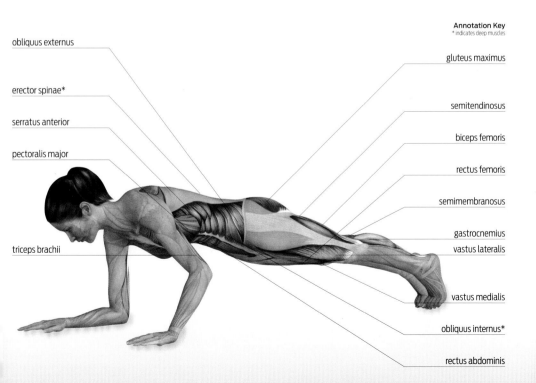

obliquus externus

erector spinae*

serratus anterior

pectoralis major

triceps brachii

gluteus maximus

semitendinosus

biceps femoris

rectus femoris

semimembranosus

gastrocnemius

vastus lateralis

vastus medialis

obliquus internus*

rectus abdominis

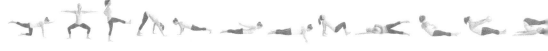

 DVD section 2: Chapter 21

Pilates Ball Tabletop–Bridge

Pilates Ball Tabletop–Bridge targets your buttocks, thighs, shoulders, and abdominals. Challenge yourself to maintain one long, straight line from your shoulders to knees while in the bridge position. Really use that ball, and you'll feel your body getting stronger and more toned.

1 Lie on your back with your arms along your sides and your legs in tabletop position with the Pilates ball between your knees.

2 Lower your feet to the mat, using your abdominals to drive the movement.

3 Press your arms into the mat for stability, engage your buttocks, and lift your pelvis so that your body from shoulders to legs forms a bridge. Use your inner-thigh muscles to hold the ball in place.

4 Stay in the bridge for a few seconds before relaxing your spine down to the mat and then returning to the tabletop position again.

5 Complete 5 repetitions.

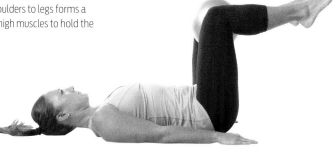

Correct form
- Keep your navel pressed toward your spine.
- Engage your buttocks, thighs, and hamstrings.
- Keep your pelvis level while in the bridge.

Avoid
- Allowing your hips to sink toward the mat.
- Arching your back while in the bridge.

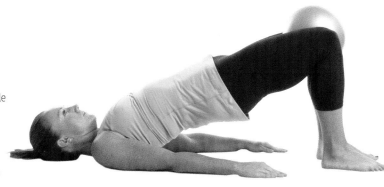

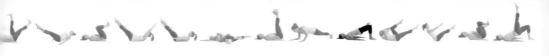

Diary of practice

	Date	Repetitions	Comment
Week 1			
Week 2			
Week 3			
Week 4			

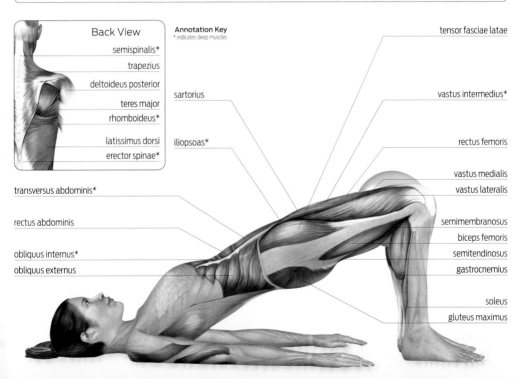

Back View

Annotation Key
* indicates deep muscles

semispinalis*
trapezius
deltoideus posterior
teres major
rhomboideus*
latissimus dorsi
erector spinae*

transversus abdominis*

rectus abdominis

obliquus internus*
obliquus externus

sartorius

iliopsoas*

tensor fasciae latae

vastus intermedius*

rectus femoris

vastus medialis
vastus lateralis

semimembranosus
biceps femoris
semitendinosus
gastrocnemius

soleus
gluteus maximus

 DVD section 2: Chapter 22

Bicycle Twists

When executing Bicycle Twists with good form, you'll get the satisfying sense that your abdominals are working hard—and getting harder in the process. Especially beneficial to the hard-to-reach obliques, these twists can be fast-paced; be sure to stay mindful of your core, engaging your abdominals throughout the entire sequence.

1 Lie on your back, with your knees bent slightly closer to your body than in tabletop position. Place your hands behind your head, and raise your upper body off the mat.

2 Extend one leg downward as far as you can go while keeping your pelvis stable and abdominals pulled in. At the same time, bring the other knee toward your chest and rotate your upper body diagonally so that your knee touches the opposite elbow.

3 Return your upper body to the center as your legs start to switch.

4 Repeat on the other side, and continue on to complete 8 to 10 full twists.

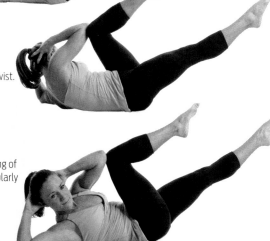

Correct form
· Touch your elbow to your opposite knee with each twist.
· Return to starting position between every twist.
· Keep your elbows wide.
· Maintain pointed feet throughout the exercise.

Avoid
· Holding your breath.
· Pushing your head with your hands; instead, the lifting of your upper body should come from your core, particularly your obliques.
· Letting your abdominals bulge outward.
· Hunching your shoulders.
· Lowering your leg so far that you arch your back.
· Racing through the exercise and sacrificing your form.

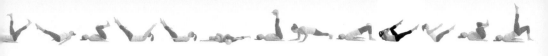

Diary of practice

	Date	Repetitions	Comment
Week 1			
Week 2			
Week 3			
Week 4			

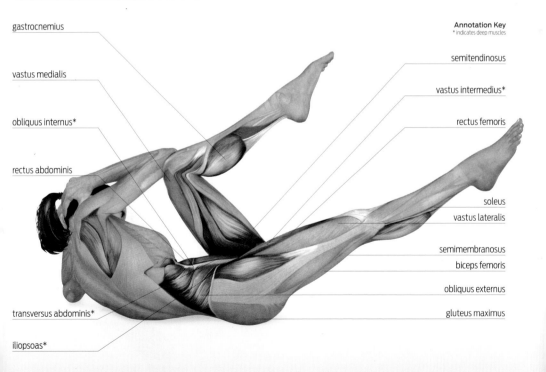

gastrocnemius

vastus medialis

obliquus internus*

rectus abdominis

transversus abdominis*

iliopsoas*

Annotation Key
* indicates deep muscles

semitendinosus

vastus intermedius*

rectus femoris

soleus

vastus lateralis

semimembranosus

biceps femoris

obliquus externus

gluteus maximus

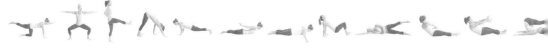

 DVD section 2: Chapter 23

Teaser Prep and Teaser

Teaser may be demanding, but it's also highly rewarding—requiring that you tune in to your body's sense of balance, strength, coordination, and alignment. Start with Teaser Prep before jumping right into this advanced move. With practice, you'll notice your abdominal strength improving dramatically.

1 To perform Teaser Prep, lie on your back with your arms extended over your head behind you. Press your bent knees together, feet flat on the mat. Straighten one leg from your hip and out through your foot.

2 Initiating the movement from your lower abdomen, raise your torso to a forward diagonal position as you bring your arms up over your head and to a forward reaching position.

3 With control, curl your spine down to the mat as you bring your arms up overhead and behind you again, keeping your knees pressed together.

4 Complete 3 repetitions on one leg before switching to the other side.

5 To start the full Teaser, lie on your back with your legs extended in front of you and your arms extended behind you.

6 As before, initiating the movement from your lower abdomen, raise your torso to a forward diagonal position. Simultaneously extend both legs forward into the space at a 45-degree angle from the mat. You are now balancing on a point a couple of inches behind your sit-bones.

7 Curl your tailbone under, press your legs firmly together, and roll down to your mat as your legs lower to the mat. Repeat 2 times.

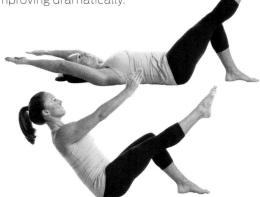

Correct form
· Keep your legs together as if they were attached.
· Keep your neck long and throat open.
· Maintain a tight core.
· Keep your pelvis level at all times.
· Initiate movement from your lower abdominals.

Avoid
· Arching your back or rolling your shoulders forward.
· Using momentum to propel yourself up and down.

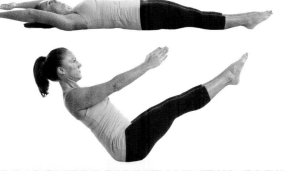

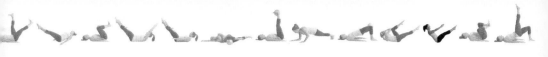

Diary of practice

	Date	Repetitions	Comment
Week 1			
Week 2			
Week 3			
Week 4			

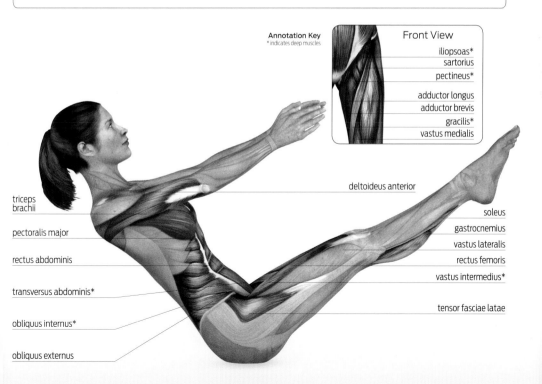

Annotation Key
* indicates deep muscles

Front View

iliopsoas*
sartorius
pectineus*
adductor longus
adductor brevis
gracilis*
vastus medialis

deltoideus anterior

triceps brachii

pectoralis major

rectus abdominis

transversus abdominis*

obliquus internus*

obliquus externus

soleus

gastrocnemius

vastus lateralis

rectus femoris

vastus intermedius*

tensor fasciae latae

 DVD section 2: Chapter 24

Frog

Frog may not be an elegant exercise, but it really targets your hip flexors and extensors—working your buttocks and abdominals along the way.

1 Lie on your back, with arms down by your sides and your legs in tabletop position. Bring your knees to a parallel closed position. Extend your spine along the mat in an imprint. Rotate your legs in your hip sockets, pressing your flexed ankles together at the heels. Your legs should be turned out.

2 Pressing your navel toward your spine, extend your turned-out legs to a 45-degree angle in the space in front of you while tightly hugging your legs together.

3 With control, draw your legs back to Frog position: legs rotated, heels together, and feet flexed.

4 Complete 6 to 10 repetitions.

Correct form
· Rotate your legs from your hip sockets.

Avoid
· Lowering your legs too far; go only as low as you can maintain complete control.
· Arching your back.
· Dropping your heels toward the mat when bringing your knees in.

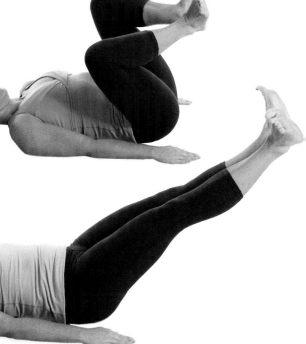

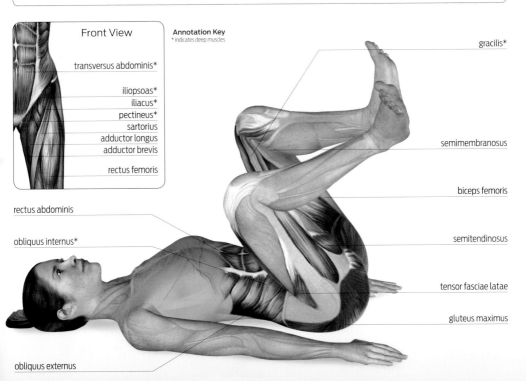

Diary of practice

	Date	Repetitions	Comment
Week 1			
Week 2			
Week 3			
Week 4			

Front View

Annotation Key
* indicates deep muscles

transversus abdominis*

iliopsoas*
iliacus*
pectineus*
sartorius
adductor longus
adductor brevis

rectus femoris

rectus abdominis

obliquus internus*

obliquus externus

gracilis*

semimembranosus

biceps femoris

semitendinosus

tensor fasciae latae

gluteus maximus

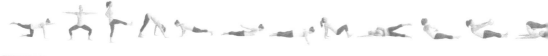

DVD section 2: Chapter 25

Single-Leg Gluteal Lift

Pilates may be known for developing sleek and strong abdominals, but the Single-Leg Gluteal Lift proves that it develops tight buttocks too. When lifting, raise your body only as high as you can go while maintaining correct alignment. If you feel strain in your lower back, you're going too far.

1 Lie on your back with your arms along your sides and legs bent with your feet directly under your knees. Extend one leg upward, pointing through your foot.

2 Engage your abdominals to pop up to a one-legged, stable bridge.

3 Maintain this position, focusing on keeping your hips level, navel pressing to spine, and free leg extending from the hip joint.

4 Lower back to the mat, keeping your leg extended.

5 Repeat to complete 5 lifts. Then, switch legs and repeat on the other side.

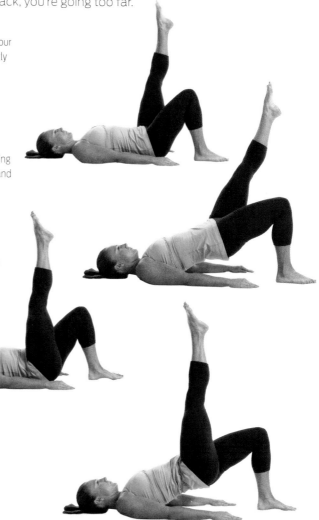

Correct form
· Engage your buttocks throughout.
· Keep your hips level at all times.
· Extend your leg out through your foot.

Avoid
· Arching your back.
· Twisting or tilting your hips while lifting.

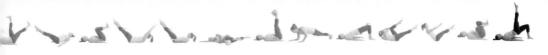

Diary of practice

	Date	Repetitions	Comment
Week 1			
Week 2			
Week 3			
Week 4			

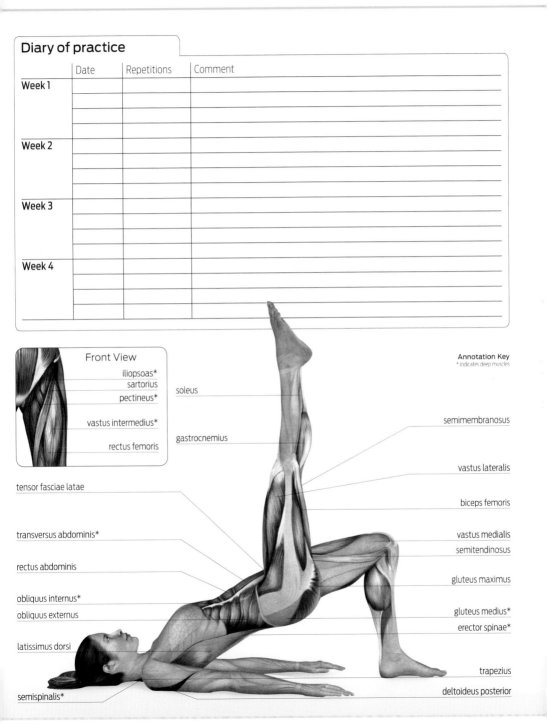

Front View

iliopsoas*
sartorius
pectineus*

vastus intermedius*

rectus femoris

soleus

gastrocnemius

tensor fasciae latae

transversus abdominis*

rectus abdominis

obliquus internus*
obliquus externus

latissimus dorsi

semispinalis*

semimembranosus

vastus lateralis

biceps femoris

vastus medialis
semitendinosus

gluteus maximus

gluteus medius*
erector spinae*

trapezius

deltoideus posterior

Full-Body Anatomy

Front View

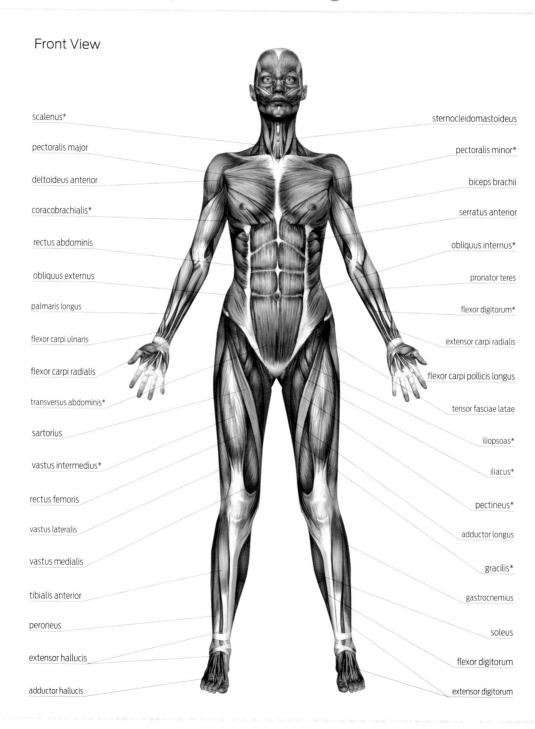

scalenus*

pectoralis major

deltoideus anterior

coracobrachialis*

rectus abdominis

obliquus externus

palmaris longus

flexor carpi ulnaris

flexor carpi radialis

transversus abdominis*

sartorius

vastus intermedius*

rectus femoris

vastus lateralis

vastus medialis

tibialis anterior

peroneus

extensor hallucis

adductor hallucis

sternocleidomastoideus

pectoralis minor*

biceps brachii

serratus anterior

obliquus internus*

pronator teres

flexor digitorum*

extensor carpi radialis

flexor carpi pollicis longus

tensor fasciae latae

iliopsoas*

iliacus*

pectineus*

adductor longus

gracilis*

gastrocnemius

soleus

flexor digitorum

extensor digitorum

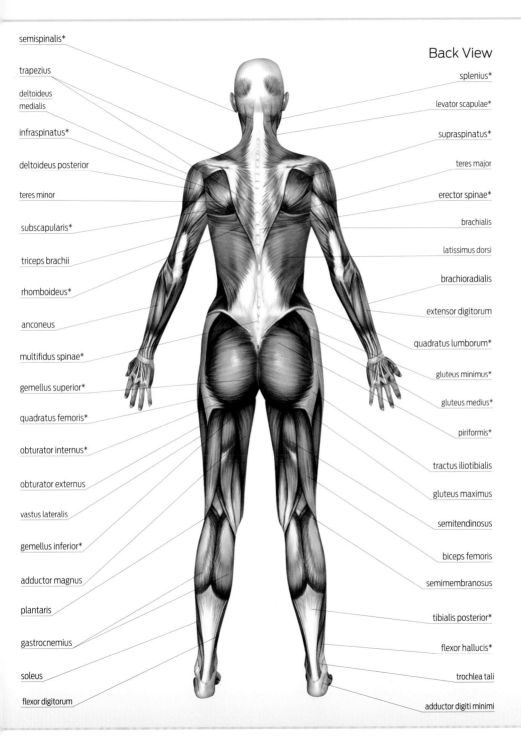

semispinalis*

trapezius

deltoideus
medialis

infraspinatus*

deltoideus posterior

teres minor

subscapularis*

triceps brachii

rhomboideus*

anconeus

multifidus spinae*

gemellus superior*

quadratus femoris*

obturator internus*

obturator externus

vastus lateralis

gemellus inferior*

adductor magnus

plantaris

gastrocnemius

soleus

flexor digitorum

Back View

splenius*

levator scapulae*

supraspinatus*

teres major

erector spinae*

brachialis

latissimus dorsi

brachioradialis

extensor digitorum

quadratus lumborum*

gluteus minimus*

gluteus medius*

piriformis*

tractus iliotibialis

gluteus maximus

semitendinosus

biceps femoris

semimembranosus

tibialis posterior*

flexor hallucis*

trochlea tali

adductor digiti minimi

Targeted Workouts

Classical Pilates Start

This series of 7 exercises gives you a sense of the progression of a traditional Pilates routine. It's certainly an excellent way to work your abdominals and move your spine, and it shouldn't require more than 10 to 15 minutes to complete. If you let one exercise flow into the next and pick up the pace, you'll be both warm and invigorated when you're finished.

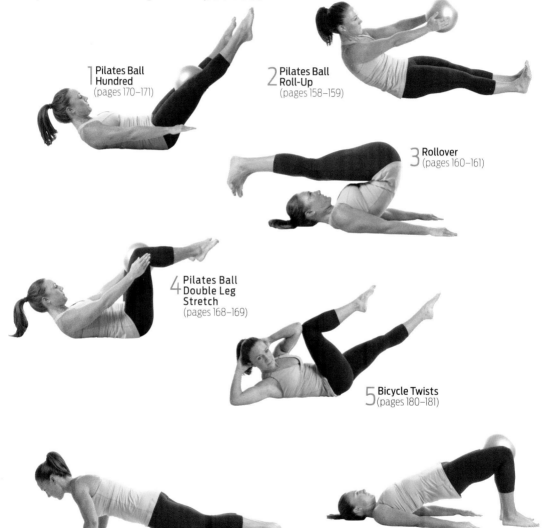

1 **Pilates Ball Hundred**
(pages 170–171)

2 **Pilates Ball Roll-Up**
(pages 158–159)

3 **Rollover**
(pages 160–161)

4 **Pilates Ball Double Leg Stretch**
(pages 168–169)

5 **Bicycle Twists**
(pages 180–181)

7 **Push-Up**
(pages 146–147)

6 **Pilates Ball Tabletop–Bridge**
(pages 178–179)

Spinal Call

This short sequence is great for energizing and re-energizing your body and mind any time during the day. Although it seems like the focus is on stretching and strengthening the spine, you'll be working those abdominals as you support every movement along the way. Notice that you start and end with the same exercise—but see how different it feels the second time around.

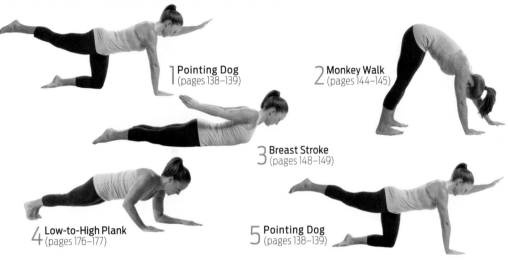

1 **Pointing Dog**
(pages 138–139)

2 **Monkey Walk**
(pages 144–145)

3 **Breast Stroke**
(pages 148–149)

4 **Low-to-High Plank**
(pages 176–177)

5 **Pointing Dog**
(pages 138–139)

Working the Leg–Core Connection

This sequence, done lying on your back or your side, automatically offers you the support of the floor to use your core to work your legs from deep in your hip sockets. The more you use your powerhouse muscles, the greater the ease of movement and power in your legs.

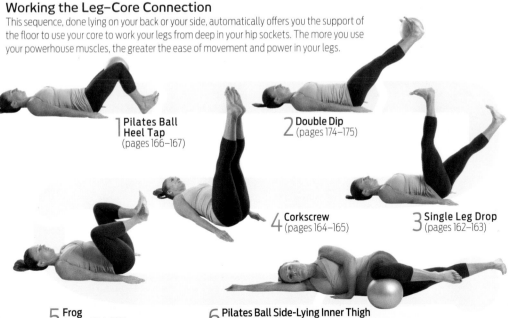

1 **Pilates Ball Heel Tap**
(pages 166–167)

2 **Double Dip**
(pages 174–175)

3 **Single Leg Drop**
(pages 162–163)

4 **Corkscrew**
(pages 164–165)

5 **Frog**
(pages 184–185)

6 **Pilates Ball Side-Lying Inner Thigh**
(pages 172–173)

About the Author

Isabel Eisen, a native New Yorker and trained dancer, lived and worked in Denmark for many years—first as a performer and then, increasingly, as an educator. She initiated and directed theater arts programs for adults and young people and was part of a group of British and Danish performing artists who established Scandinavian Theatre School in Copenhagen. She wrote a book, *Danseværksted,* and articles about her teaching ideas and practice, which were published in Denmark. Her deep involvement in teaching, coupled with her interest in intelligent exercising, led her to Pilates, which she studied intensively for several years at Body Control and Stott Pilates studios in Denmark. In 2010, Ms. Eisen returned to New York City, where she continues to pursue her work with teaching, writing, and Pilates.

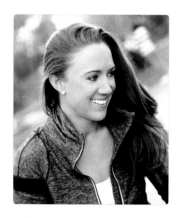

Pilates model and consultant Brooke Marrone turned her successful collegiate pursuits into a thriving full-time career as a fitness trainer. Her post-graduation experience studying under one of Boston's top trainers formed the basis for the safe and effective training philosophy that she follows today. In 2007, Brooke moved to New York City and started Brooke Marrone Fitness, a private, in-home training business. Brooke also hosts group classes in New York's Central Park and has been named an ambassador for Lululemon in both 2011 and 2012. Brooke's certifications include Personal Training, Pilates and Group Fitness. Brooke's training strategy is to stick to the basics while always trying to incorporate something new and unique into each workout. She integrates her personal training and Pilates knowledge to make each workout safe, creative, and challenging.

hinkler

Published by Hinkler Books Pty Ltd 2014
45–55 Fairchild Street
Heatherton Victoria 3202 Australia
www.hinkler.com.au

Copyright © Hinkler Books Pty Ltd 2012, 2014

ISBN: 978 1 7436 3860 6